D0960409

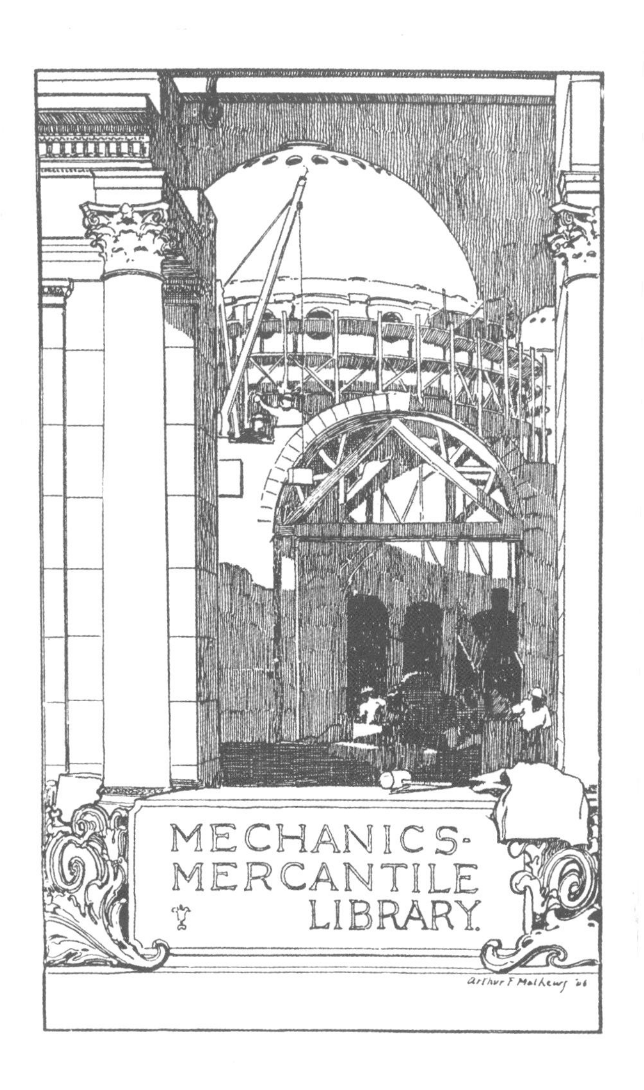
MECHANICS-
MERCANTILE
LIBRARY.
Arthur F Mathews '06

Medicine by Design

Medicine by Design

The Practice and Promise of Biomedical Engineering

FEN MONTAIGNE

THE JOHNS HOPKINS UNIVERSITY PRESS
Baltimore

Printed in the United States of America on acid-free paper
9 8 7 6 5 4 3 2 1

The Johns Hopkins University Press
2715 North Charles Street
Baltimore, Maryland 21218-4363
www.press.jhu.edu

Library of Congress Cataloging-in-Publication Data

Montaigne, Fen.
Medicine by design : the practice and promise of biomedical engineering / Fen Montaigne.
p. ; cm.
Includes index.
ISBN 0-8018-8347-4 (hardcover : alk. paper)
1. Biomedical engineering. I. Title.
[DNLM: 1. Biomedical Engineering—Trends—Case Reports.
2. Biomedical Engineering—Trends—Popular Works. QT 36 M761m 2006]
R856. M595 2006
610'.29—dc22 2005021214

A catalog record for this book is available from the British Library.

To my father-in-law,
Dr. Richard M. Hays—

brilliant researcher,
compassionate physician,
marvelous grandfather,
and loving father

Contents

Acknowledgments

I am deeply indebted to the many biomedical engineers, physicians, scientists, and students who met with me as I traveled around the country researching this book. Biomedical engineering is a new, sprawling, and complex field, and were it not for the hospitality and patience of the more than 200 people I interviewed, I would never have been able to pull off this project. I am especially indebted to the following people: Shu Chien, chairman of the Bioengineering Department at the University of California, San Diego; Katherine W. Ferrara, founding chairwoman of the Department of Biomedical Engineering at the University of California, Davis; Kenneth R. Lutchen, chairman of the Department of Biomedical Engineering at Boston University; Robert M. Nerem, director of the Georgia Tech / Emory Center for the Engineering of Living Tissues; P. Hunter Peckham, executive director of the Cleveland FES Center and professor of biomedical engineering at Case University; Clinton R. Rubin, chairman of the Department of Biomedical Engineering at the State University of New York, Stony Brook; Thomas C. Skalak, chairman of the Department of Biomedical Engineering at the University of Virginia; and Savior L.-Y. Woo, director of the Musculoskeletal Research Center at the University of Pittsburgh. And for all their help I also would like to thank Michael Lysaght, director of Brown University's Center for Biomedical Engineering, and Martin L. Yarmush, chairman of the Department of Biomedical Engineering at Rutgers University.

I want to thank Mary Buckett of the Cleveland FES Center for her kind assistance. Thanks, as well, to Claudia Morain of the UC Davis Cancer Center. I am also indebted to Earl Bakken and all the people at Medtronic who met with me, and thanks to Medtronic's Christine

Campbell-Loth and Richard Fischer for helping arrange my visits to the company's headquarters. I also want to thank Weng Tao and her colleagues at Neurotech for speaking with me about their company.

I am also grateful to the dozens of patients who took the time to speak with me about their lives and how biomedical engineering had changed them. Thanks to you all.

This book would not have come into being without the support and financial underwriting of the Whitaker Foundation, which is fitting, since the field of biomedical engineering would not be where it is today without the foundation's generosity and unstinting efforts. The foundation has done more than any single private organization to foster the growth of biomedical engineering as an academic discipline. In the course of three decades, the foundation spent more than $900 million, most of it to help create and build new departments of biomedical engineering or expand existing ones. It also supported the research of more than 1,000 engineers and scientists. In its relatively brief life, the foundation had a unique impact on biomedical engineering, a discipline that has made great contributions to improving human health. This impact was possible because of the foundation's decision to close its doors, in line with the wishes of U. A. Whitaker, whose fortune was used to establish the foundation in the early 1970s. Because of its decision to spend all of its funds, the foundation was able to shape a field in a way that few other nonprofit groups have ever done. The departments of biomedical engineering I visited for this book all benefited from the foundation's generosity. The foundation will cease to exist in the summer of 2006, but its legacy will live on for decades.

I am indebted to the foundation's governing committee and would particularly like to thank chairman G. Burtt Holmes and U. A. Whitaker's daughters, Ruth Whitaker Holmes and Portia Whitaker Shumaker. The committee's staff also was extremely helpful throughout, and I would particularly like to thank Frank N. Blanchard, Mark A. Bowman, James A. Frost, Peter G. Katona, and John H. Linehan.

Many thanks to my literary agent, Michael Carlisle, for his continued support and his important role in this project. Thanks to Vincent J. Burke, my editor at the Johns Hopkins University Press, for his many valuable ideas and his thoughtful work on the manuscript. Thanks also to Grace Carino for her fine job copyediting this work.

Finally, I would like to thank my wife, Laurie Hays, and my daughters, Claire and Nuni, for their understanding, patience, and love as yet another assignment took me away from home. And many thanks to my father-in-law, Dr. Richard M. Hays, whose kind soul and decades of medical knowledge were invaluable as I wrote this book.

Medicine by Design

Prologue

Whether Jay Joyce would be a dead man today without biomedical engineering, or merely a very unhappy one, is open to debate. But one thing is certain. Were it not for the implantable cardiac defibrillator in his chest, Jay Joyce would lead a far different life, assuming he had one to live at all.

A West Point graduate and former army officer who had completed Airborne Ranger training, Joyce was 46 years old when he discovered that he was afflicted with a rare and potentially fatal heart ailment. He learned of this quirk in his anatomy on an icy, overcast day in late December 1998 when, after jogging 15 miles, he returned home to discover that his body was in the process of betraying him. Normally, when the supremely fit Joyce did stretching exercises after a long run, his heart rate would settle down from about 125 beats per minute to 60. But on this day, his heart rate went in the opposite direction and stayed there. For five hours, his heart beat 200 times per minute, a condition known as tachycardia. He felt short of breath and vomited when he tried to eat. Being a former army officer, Joyce thought he could tough out a situation that would have sent most people to the emergency room hours before.

"I really felt like hell," recalled Joyce, a trim man with dark, receding hair and a mustache. "All I did was sit on the sofa and sip water."

Finally, as his rapid heartbeat continued into the sixth hour, he agreed to go to the hospital. There, he underwent the usual ritual of processing and triage, until a doctor put a stethoscope to his chest. "Everything in the ER stopped," Joyce recalled, "and I became the center of attention."

His electrocardiogram resembled a seismograph during an earthquake. His pulse was now over 200 beats per minute, his heart pounding so rapidly, Joyce remembered, "that my body was literally rocking back and forth." Doctors administered drugs to bring his heart rate down, and Joyce began to feel better. He was released from the emergency room that day. But that was only the start of what Joyce calls his "cardiac journey," an odyssey that ended when the former soldier received one of the most elegant inventions produced by the marriage of engineering and medicine: the implantable cardiac defibrillator.

Joyce—an executive at a major consumer products company and the father of two children who also have served in the U.S. Army—set out to find what was ailing him. He did not have to go far. Near his home in Norwich, New York, Joyce was fortunate to find a first-rate cardiac electrophysiologist, Dr. Nicholas Stamato. Using a variety of tools created by the collaboration of doctors and engineers—electrical mapping of the heart using catheters inserted into arteries, and magnetic resonance imaging (MRI) to obtain detailed, three-dimensional images of the beating organ—Stamato was able to make a diagnosis. Joyce had a rare condition, affecting about 1 in 5,000 people, known as arrhythmogenic right ventricular dysplasia (ARVD). It is a genetic, progressive disease in which the muscle in the heart's right ventricle turns into fatty or fibrous tissue, interfering with the conduction of electrical signals that make the heart beat regularly. The MRI showed that Joyce's right ventricle had distended to more than twice its normal size, as the diseased tissue had slowly ballooned. And, Stamato said, it would only get worse.

The condition often leads to the tachycardia Joyce had experienced. And ARVD tachycardia can easily turn into ventricular fibrillation, a deadly condition in which the cardiac muscle descends into a chaotic, quivering state, beating several hundred times a minute. With the heart unable to pump blood, people in ventricular fibrillation lose consciousness in fifteen to twenty seconds. Left untreated, they die in several minutes. ARVD and related conditions have led to the sudden deaths of young athletes in recent years, including the college basketball player Hank Gaithers.

Stamato told Joyce there was a solution to his problem: the implantable defibrillator. On the market for twenty years, the defibrillator senses when the heart is in fibrillation and administers a powerful shock that resets the heart and restores a normal heart rhythm. After obtaining a second opinion from the University of Pennsylvania, where doctors confirmed the diagnosis, Joyce decided to have Stamato implant the device.

On February 24, 1999, Joyce went to the Wilson Memorial Regional Medical Center in Johnson City, New York. With Joyce under short-term anesthesia, Stamato made a 4-inch incision in the upper-left chest, just below the collarbone. He inserted a stopwatch-sized defibrillator made by Medtronic, the country's leading manufacturer of cardiac pacemakers and other implantable medical devices. Stamato ran two leads from the defibrillator to Joyce's heart through a major blood vessel. He then anchored the leads into Joyce's heart muscle.

After implanting the device, Stamato tested it by stimulating the heart into tachycardia and then seeing whether the defibrillator detected the rapid heartbeat and administered a shock. Most patients choose to remain asleep during the test, but Joyce had other ideas.

"I had done a lot of research and I knew that the single biggest anxiety people have about the defibrillator is, 'What does this thing feel like when it goes off inside me?'" said Joyce. "Anxiety stems from the unknown and I wanted to know. I told Dr. Stamato I wanted to be awake and he looked at me like I was crazy.

"He explained to me what he was going to do. I could feel my heart starting to race and he said, 'Here it comes,' and I swear, I was strapped down and I still jumped three inches off that table. I tend to describe it as like putting each of your index fingers in a socket for a second. It's not painful, but man is it a jolt! But the neat thing about it is that after that, at least I knew what it was like."

With a new device in his chest, Joyce set about resuming his old life. Doctors believe that exercise can trigger tachycardia and ventricular fibrillation in people with ARVD. But Joyce was not about to stop running or leading an active life. Stamato realized that slowing Joyce down would be hard and, after spelling out the increased risks from exercise, advised him to take it slowly. Joyce agreed, but his attitude was, "Look, you've got to understand. I am not sick. I hate to be referred to as a patient."

By that July, just five months after the defibrillator was implanted, Joyce completed the 9.3-mile Boilermaker run in Utica, New York, a feat he repeated in ensuing years. He jogged nearly as much as he had before, and on four occasions during exercise the defibrillator zapped him as his heart accelerated to a dangerously high rate. On one occasion he was jogging with his son, also a West Point graduate.

"When it went off he was scared to death because I jumped a lot," recalled Joyce. "He said, 'Dad, we've got to go home.' But we just walked awhile and I was okay. When this thing fires, I stand there a few seconds and then I start running again. It's like a TV signal getting scrambled and then unscrambled, and then you're just fine. I wouldn't use the word *painful* to describe the shock. It's more a matter that it's grossly uncomfortable."

On another occasion, he was on a treadmill at a gym when the defibrillator kicked into action. The jolt propelled him nearly off the treadmill, causing him to stumble and crash to the ground.

Joyce, who now lives in Cincinnati, views the shocks as a small price to pay for living the life he wants to lead. In all likelihood, the device has saved his life, for his condition is worsening and it was only a matter of time before his tachycardia turned into a fatal episode of ventricular fibrillation. In March 2005, he received a new version of Medtronic's defibrillator, one designed to bring the heart out of severe tachycardia or fibrillation by first issuing a number of imperceptible charges, a technique known as pacing the heart out of a severe arrhythmia. If the pacing fails, the defibrillator will unleash a shock. But Joyce doesn't dwell on the prospect. Indeed, when his defibrillator fires, it is a reminder that he carries inside him a tiny machine that has the power to save his life.

For a field that few people have heard of and even fewer understand, biomedical engineering has come to the rescue of an awful lot of us. If you're healthy and have never spent a day in a hospital, then you may have managed to avoid coming into contact with the devices and treatments that are the hallmark of biomedical engineering. Otherwise you have no doubt benefited from a field that didn't even exist half a century ago but that, along with the pharmaceutical industry and the spread of vaccines, has saved and improved an enormous number of lives in recent decades. Every person with a pacemaker, a defibrillator, or an artificial joint has tasted the fruits of biomedical engineering. Anyone who has had an MRI or a computerized tomography (CT) scan, who has had an artery propped open with a stent, or who has been kept alive during coronary artery bypass surgery with a heart-lung machine, likewise has been served by biomedical engineering. Wounded soldiers with artificial limbs, people who have had their blood automatically analyzed by machine, diabetics with portable, pager-sized insulin pumps, and people with Parkinson's disease who have had their tremors stilled by implanted electrodes—all have been aided by biomedical engineering.

What is this field? At its simplest level, it is the union of engineering and medicine to improve health care. For a couple of decades in the mid-twentieth century, it was not even a recognized discipline but rather was the domain of engineers, doctors, and physicists who invented, tinkered with, and cobbled together devices that never before existed. The pioneers were people like Earl Bakken, the founder of Medtronic, who made the first battery-powered, transistorized pacemaker; Wilhelm Kolff, a Dutchman who invented the first kidney dialysis machine; and John Gibbon, a Philadelphia physician who made the first machine that could oxygenate a patient's blood while the heart was stopped for cardiac surgery.

Over three decades, starting in the 1960s, these scattered areas of endeavor began to be recognized as a unified discipline, one in which the traditional methods of engineering—the application of mathematics, modeling, and the use of electrical, chemical, and mechanical systems to break down and solve problems—could be brought to bear on medicine. Today, the field has evolved to the point where roughly seventy-five universities have created departments of biomedical engineering, their goal being to produce students steeped in the basics of engineering and physiology.

In this new century, biomedical engineering is inevitably shifting its focus from inventing devices to exploring science's most alluring terrain: the cell and the genome. Biomedical engineers are aiming their analytical weapons at the building blocks of life. Using their ability to crunch huge quantities of data with supercomputers and to analyze problems in a systematic way, biomedical engineers are studying how vast networks of genes interact to create the proteins that make up human physiology and disease. They are probing the workings of the cell in order to one day build tissue, and perhaps even organs, in the lab. They are exploring the intricate domain of the brain, in the hope of using genetic engineering, electrical stimulation, or even tiny machines to treat devastating diseases such as Alzheimer's and Parkinson's.

This book is a journey across the fascinating landscape of biomedical engineering. It takes readers into the universities and companies where engineers, doctors, and other scientists are quietly doing the work that is revolutionizing health care. Above all, this is a story about people—people who are devoting their lives to tackling the medical challenges of the twenty-first century, and people who have benefited from that labor.

Jay Joyce is one of those people, and his experience has given him an appreciation for the small army of engineers and scientists he scarcely knew existed.

"I am convinced that I might well not be alive if I didn't have the defibrillator," said Joyce. "Look what this technology has enabled me to do. I believe I will live to be 70 or 80 and I'll be a young 70 or 80. There's a perception out there that people who get these devices are sick old people. But the real benefit of something like the defibrillator is that we can take a healthy 46-year-old guy with a medical problem and make him a contributor to society for the next forty years."

Chapter 1

The Rise of a New Field

On a cool, sunny, spring morning, about 200 people gathered in an auditorium at Boston University's Photonics Center, just a few blocks from the Charles River. They had assembled for what has become a rite of passage for biomedical engineering students at BU: the senior class presentation of the projects they had labored on during the academic year. Among those present were representatives from fifty companies and hospitals, as well as dozens of faculty, graduate students, and alumni. Then there were the seniors themselves, fifty-nine young men and women who had spent the past several weeks in a sleep-starved marathon as they put the finishing touches on scientific investigations ranging from how to build artificial blood vessels to manipulating genes in human cells.

The seniors were a diverse group—including students from China, India, Palestine, and Russia—and roughly half were women. They also were almost unrecognizable to anyone who had seen them during the past few weeks. Gone were the blue jeans and baseball caps, replaced by dark suits for the men and dresses and pantsuits for the women. As the seniors filed into the auditorium, one of their professors, Irving J. Bigio, remarked, "They clean up well, don't they?"

Running the show was Ken Lutchen, the longtime chairman of Boston University's Department of Biomedical Engineering and the person most responsible for making the senior project a cornerstone of his students' education. Under Lutchen's guidance, BU has developed one of the most comprehensive biomedical engineering programs in the country, giving its students a solid grounding in basic engineering studies during the first two years, then offering a wide variety of courses—such as tissue engineering and imaging—during the final two years. But Lutchen was most proud of the twenty-year tradition of the senior project, begun in the mid-1980s, which requires students to spend months working on an unsolved problem in biomedical engineering.

"I think this is the most crucial component of their education," Lutchen said a few days before the conference. "One of the main goals is to teach them how to tackle an insurmountable problem and give them confidence. During the senior year we break them down in the early stages of the project, then we build them up, and at the end they're so proud. It teaches them that they can get out in the world and succeed."

In his opening remarks, Lutchen introduced himself as the chair of the department and "torturer of the students," and he then urged the faculty and industry representatives to expose the students to withering questioning.

"My advice," said Lutchen, "is to let them have it."

The final student to take the stage during the morning session was Valmeek Kudesia, known as Vick. Kudesia not only was majoring in biomedical engineering but also was among an elite group of BU undergraduates accepted early into the medical school, where he already was taking some classes. After earning his medical degree, Kudesia's goal is to straddle the worlds of engineering and medicine and invent devices to treat heart disease. Indeed, for his senior project, Kudesia had devised an elaborate computer program to simulate a new electrode that could be used to shock a fibrillating heart back into rhythm.

A stocky man with dark hair and a dry sense of humor, Kudesia explained ventricular fibrillation—the rapid, chaotic, and often fatal misfiring of the heart—to his audience. Then he showed a computer simulation of the disorder.

"This is ventricular fibrillation, and this is ugly," he said, drawing the first laugh of the morning.

Kudesia went on to describe a commonly used implantable defibrillator, Medtronic's Cardioverter, which nearly always succeeds in restoring a rhythmic beat by delivering a powerful shock to the heart. Kudesia's goal, he explained, was to create a computer model of a new device, known as a focal defibrillator, that would restore heart rhythm with a far less powerful shock. Over the course of many months and numerous computer simulations, Kudesia came up with a new cross-shaped design that, by being placed strategically atop the damaged heart muscle that often kicks off ventricular fibrillation, would theoretically act more efficiently than conventional defibrillators.

He flashed a slide on a screen showing a model of a fibrillating heart, followed by a model of the heart receiving a jolt from his focal defibrillator.

"Two, one—bam!" he called out, drawing more laughs from the audience as his computer-simulated heart got back on track.

"This results in a less painful shock and in less battery use," Kudesia told the conference. "There's almost a magical decrease (in electricity use), and engineers don't do magic. The next step would be to do a 3-D model and more simulations that are more like reality. Far off would be to test the device in a sheep's cardiac muscle. We also need to find software to better identify scar tissue on the heart."

At the end of Kudesia's eight-minute presentation, the audience responded with enthusiastic applause. Numerous people raised their hands with questions, including Professor Bigio. Kudesia was about to respond when Lutchen fired off another question.

"My question first," Bigio joked.

"Well," replied Kudesia, smiling at Lutchen, "he controls my grade."

The audience asked a handful of questions before the lunch break, with some probing into how well the model would actually work in practice. The crowd was plainly impressed, however, that a 21-year-old had succeeded in pulling off one of the most important exercises in biomedical engineering: applying engineering techniques, including inventive computer modeling, to tackle a major medical problem.

For the BU students in the audience, the dozens of elaborate research projects presented over the course of ten hours seemed impressive but hardly extraordinary. After all, they had matriculated to a university with a well-established degree program in biomedical engineering. They listened to lectures and did laboratory work in new buildings specially constructed to house biomedical engineers, as well as scientists working with the human genome. Many of their grandparents, and even some of their parents, were kept alive with biomedical engineering hardware—pacemakers, stents, defibrillators—and when someone fell seriously ill, chances were good they would make a pass through an engineering marvel like an MRI machine or CT scanner. One of the students, a diabetic, wore an external pump that dispensed insulin into his bloodstream. For these students, born after 1980, engineering and medicine seemed a natural fit, and they were scarcely surprised that their classmates had spent their final year in college working on research projects that, only two decades before, would have represented unimaginable terrain for undergraduate students to explore.

But to an older person with experience in medicine and engineering, the scene that day in the Boston University auditorium would have seemed remarkable. Just fifty years earlier, no clearly defined field of biomedical engineering existed, and the techniques of mechanical and electrical engineering were only beginning to be applied to medicine and human health. Heart pacemakers were just being developed, artificial hips and joints were not yet being implanted, and the only way of seeing inside the human body was with an X-ray machine. If you had a persistent pain in your abdomen, a doctor attempting to figure out what was wrong would likely cut you open and take a look. And not one American university had established a curriculum or degree program in which engineering students were trained to bring their profession's skills to bear on human health.

In the 1950s and 1960s, a small number of visionaries saw the need to merge engineering and medicine for the benefit of humanity. One of the most prominent was Uncas Aeneas Whitaker, an unassuming engineer and businessman who had made his fortune developing solderless connections to join wires to electrical terminals in cars, boats, planes, computers, and household appliances. In the 1950s, he began donating money to encourage biomedical engineering research at institutions like the Massachusetts Institute of Technology (MIT) and the Cleveland Clinic. And before his death in 1975, he requested that the bulk of his estate—which then totaled roughly $100 million—be used to further expand the reach of engineering into health care.

In the ensuing thirty years, the nonprofit organization he and his wife created, the Whitaker Foundation, has done more than any other private group to fund research in biomedical engineering and establish biomedical engineering as a formal discipline at American universities. The foundation has given away money totaling nine times Whitaker's original bequest and has been instrumental in creating and expanding biomedical engineering departments on college campuses throughout the United States. When the Whitaker Foundation came into being three decades ago, only a handful of universities had biomedical engineering programs. Today, seventy-three American universities have full-fledged departments of biomedical engineering, and another forty-three engineering schools offer an undergraduate major in the field. Boston University now has one of the largest biomedical engineering departments in the country, with 33 faculty, 350 undergraduates, and 130 graduate students.

The recent, rapid expansion of biomedical engineering departments at Boston University, the Johns Hopkins University, the University of California at San Diego, and numerous other universities was spurred by major grants from the Whitaker Foundation. It also financially supported the research of 1,300 investigators. Much of the foundation's impact was due to its decision, made in the early 1990s, to take the rare step of closing its doors in 2006, in keeping with U. A. Whitaker's wish that the foundation cease to exist within forty years of his death.

By spending its capital and infusing large sums of money into biomedical engineering in a short period of time, the foundation was able to jump-start the field. Dozens of researchers around the country acknowledged that Whitaker's investment in biomedical engineering departments has played the pivotal role in launching a discipline that will be at the center of important medical breakthroughs in the twenty-first century.

"The Whitaker Foundation literally made the field of biomedical engineering what it is today," said Shu Chien, chairman of the Bioengineering Department at the University of California, San Diego.

Lawrence Schramm, a professor of biomedical engineering and the history of science at Johns Hopkins, said, "The Whitaker Foundation has expanded the reach of biomedical engineering into so many universities. They have set a standard for research and education in biomedical engineering that is so high that I think it will reverberate for a long, long time. Their insistence on high quality has contributed to this field in a very special way. I don't know what they thought they would do, but they never dreamed they would do this much. The decision to spend themselves out of business was very important. They felt they couldn't make enough of an impact if they just spent their earnings. They saw it as the time to get biomedical engineering going. It was absolutely brilliant. They have given this field a kick-start that no other field has had."

Uncas Whitaker could scarcely have imagined what his fortune would accomplish.

Born in rural Missouri in 1900, the son of a prosperous farmer who also served in the state legislature, Uncas Whitaker personified the American century. Growing up in the small town of Weaubleau, Missouri, he was infected by the excitement that surrounded the spread of the technological and industrial marvels of the early twentieth century: the car, the airplane, and the radio. Named for one of the heroes in James Fenimore Cooper's *The Last of the Mohicans,* Uncas Whitaker was fascinated by the inner workings of the machines that surrounded him. In high school he spent hours tinkering with an old Model T, and he developed a passion for aviation that would continue through his life.

Whitaker went east to MIT and earned a degree in mechanical engineering. As his biographer W. H. Cohn has pointed out, he had a highly practical bent. For his senior thesis, he designed a machine to test rubber heels so shoe companies could determine how quickly their products would wear out.

Graduating in 1923, Whitaker spent the next eighteen years rising rapidly through the ranks of several industrial corporations, working as director of research and design for the Hoover vacuum company and the American Machine and Foundry Company. He earned another degree, this one in electrical engineering from Carnegie Tech in Pittsburgh, which eventually became Carnegie Mellon University. But he was anxious to run his own business, and in 1941 he found what he was looking for: the opportunity to invest in and run an existing, small company that performed the unglamorous task of attaching electrical wires to terminals in boats and planes.

Whitaker's acquisition turned out to be a brilliant move. First, he realized that the method most companies were using to attach wires to electrical terminals—by soldering them—was primitive and unreliable. Exposed to the battering that planes and boats took, the connections often broke loose, knocking out parts of the electrical systems. Whitaker, who believed in the inevitable triumph of the reliable, well-engineered solution, helped invent and refine a better idea: a crimper—first applied by hand and later by machine—that rapidly and efficiently formed a far stronger connection between wires and terminals.

Whitaker came up with this innovation at a propitious time, just as America's industrial machine was gearing up for war against Germany and Japan. Soon, the boats and planes being mass-produced for the war effort contained Uncas Whitaker's patented crimped wires. The company, called Aircraft-Marine Products, Inc., or AMP, grew rapidly during the war. When peace came in 1945, AMP then rode the wave of America's industrial prosperity throughout the globe, eventually producing the electrical connections for everything from BMW sedans, to IBM computers, to Japanese electronics. With plants around the United States and the world, AMP rapidly occupied a place in the middle of *Fortune* magazine's top 500 American corporations. The company enjoyed 15 percent growth a year, and by 2000 Uncas Whitaker's once obscure firm had $5.7 billion in sales and 46,500 workers in more than fifty countries.

Through it all, Whitaker—a quiet man with a keen intellect—lived a modest existence. He didn't marry until he was 44 years old, and two years later, when his sister died, he adopted her daughters—Ruth, 13, and Portia, 11. Despite his wealth, the family lived in a three-bedroom home near AMP's headquarters in Harrisburg, Pennsylania. At lunchtime, he would eat at a nearby Howard Johnson's restaurant, talking with his employees at the counter. After acquiring AMP, he didn't take a vacation for ten years. He had one indulgence, sailing, and eventually bought a sailboat and a summer home on Swan's Island, Maine.

At home, he and his wife read classics to Ruth and Portia at night. He also enjoyed reading aloud Frank Galbraith's *Cheaper by the Dozen.* Like the hero of that memoir, he was concerned about domestic efficiency, even keeping a daily journal that logged, among other things, how much time it took him to shave (two and a half minutes). He was concerned that his adopted daughters not become spoiled by his wealth, and as they grew, he cautioned them that he planned to give away most of his fortune. Before teaching Ruth how to drive, he first taught her how to fix a flat. When she left for college, he gave her a toolkit.

In the 1950s and 1960s, as Whitaker took stock of all that he had accomplished, he felt that one important piece of business remained unfinished. As he came in more frequent contact with America's hospitals and health care system—his sister had died of cancer, and Whitaker himself had had a series of heart attacks in the early 1960s—he was surprised by how little the medical profession was benefiting from engineering. He believed that science and engineering could solve almost any problem, and he dedicated himself to an overriding goal: to do everything he could to encourage engineers to use their skills to improve medical care.

"He was the consummate engineer and he believed engineering

was the solution to darned near everything," recalled Miles J. Gibbons Jr., who worked as an attorney for AMP and later served as president of the Whitaker Foundation. "His whole life was based on engineering, he recognized how little engineering was being used in medicine, and he was drawn to do something about that."

Dr. George Thorn, a renowned Boston physician who served with Whitaker on MIT's board of trustees and helped him shape his early ideas about biomedical engineering research, recalled that Whitaker was one of a small number of engineers who had the vision to see what the profession could do for health care.

"In our talks, he would point out what a great opportunity there was for engineering to take its rightful place in medical advances," Thorn told me a few months before his death, at the age of 98, in 2004. "The timing was just right."

In the late 1950s, Whitaker funded several biomedical engineering research projects at MIT, and later he gave $2.1 million to help build the Uncas A. and Helen F. Whitaker Building for the Life Sciences at MIT. He was the driving force behind the creation of the joint Harvard-MIT Program in Health Sciences and Technology, which supported biomedical engineering projects and trained students in biomedical engineering. In addition, he endowed a program to encourage collaboration between MIT and medical schools at Harvard, Tufts, and Boston University. At the same time, Whitaker helped establish a program at the Cleveland Clinic that provided information and treatment to people with cardiovascular disease.

"He was light years ahead of other people in seeing the need to bring engineering and the basic sciences into health care," said G. Burtt Holmes, Whitaker's son-in-law and the longtime chairman of the Whitaker Foundation. "Everybody talks that way today. But when he talked about it in the 1940s and 50s he was almost like a lone voice in the wilderness. He was a pioneer."

Whitaker's interest in fostering the growth of biomedical engineering came at a time when the field was poised to take off and change the way medicine was practiced. Prior to 1950, physicians had very few devices and diagnostic tools at their disposal. There was the microscope, the X-ray machine, the blood-pressure cuff, electrocardiograms (ECG) to analyze heart function, and implements for surgery. Until 1961, when the University of Pennsylvania created America's first department of biomedical engineering, there was, in effect, no official union between medicine and engineering. Indeed, in the 1950s and 1960s, many doctors tended to look down upon engineers who dabbled in medicine, and many engineers thought that their colleagues working in the medical world had gone astray. The term *biomedical engineer* conjured up visions of someone repairing machines in hospitals rather than inventing new medical technologies.

But in the decades after World War II, the hard science of engineering began to move into the field of medicine, and with spectacular results. Many of the pioneers in biomedical engineering were people like Whitaker, inventors with an unshakable belief that even the human body could be fixed by engineering. In America, in the 1950s, inventors and physicians such as Paul M. Zoll, Dr. C. Walton Lillehei, Earl Bakken, William M. Chardack, and Wilson Greatbatch invented heart pacemakers and the batteries to eventually make them fully implantable. Also in the 1950s, electrical engineer Wallace Coulter invented a device that has revolutionized medicine: the Coulter Counter, which enables machines to analyze blood rapidly and accurately.

But the real transformation of biomedical engineering came with the computer revolution of the 1960s. Computers were able to crunch more data than anyone ever dreamed possible, a breakthrough that was vital to the rise of new types of imaging, such as MRI and CT, both of which began to be used clinically in the 1980s. It was computing power that eventually opened the way to decoding the genetic secrets of living organisms, a fertile new field for biomedical engineers.

Today, it is impossible to imagine the high standard of medical care in the developed world without the contributions of biomedical engineering. Michael Lysaght, director of the Center for Biomedical Engineering at Brown University, says the "three D's"—devices, drugs, and diagnostics—have revolutionized medical care in the United States and the industrialized world. Biomedical engineers have played a vital role in engineering new devices and diagnostic tools, and engineering advances have been instrumental in enabling pharmaceutical companies to test thousands of compounds a day in the search for new drugs.

Take a look at family and friends and it becomes evident how crucial biomedical engineering has been in extending average life expectancy in the United States from 47 in 1900 to 77 today. Who doesn't know someone whose life has been saved or bettered by a biomedical engineering device, such as a pacemaker? All these lifesaving and life-extending machines and surgical procedures cost money, however, and lots of it. A century ago, America spent only 2 percent of its gross national product on health care. By 1960, that figure was 6 percent. Today it is 15 percent, and in another decade or two it is likely to hit 20 percent. The need to control rising medical costs is a pressing one, but who would deny a parent or sibling medical procedures, such as a heart bypass operation, that could give them twenty more years of life?

"Anything that extends life increases health care costs," said Lysaght. "But in a free society it's difficult to find a better target than providing people with more longevity and better health care. Scientists like to measure end points and the easiest end point to measure in medicine and health care is death. Life expectancy is 77 today and each recent generation has had a life span six years longer than the previous generation. Health care used to be cheap because medical knowledge was limited. Now we can do wondrous things but you pay for it. And biomedical engineering has contributed in a major way."

Lysaght sees no slowdown either in the battle to continue extending the time we spend on earth or in rising health care costs.

"One of the dominant factors in the next 50 years is going to be the aging of society," said Lysaght. "People will continue to live longer simply because health care is better. You will see a large portion of health care resources being spent on keeping people healthier for the full length of their life. Scientists are going to be extending our life span by going in and altering what it is that causes people to die. You want to compress the morbidity at the end. Ronald Reagan [who died a lingering death from Alzheimer's disease] is an example of what you don't want to happen. Kate Hepburn [who remained vibrant to the end] is."

Chapter 2

The New Generation

Vick Kudesia and his classmate Inas Khayal were among the best of a very good lot at Boston University. Both immigrated to the United States at a young age, both were drawn to BU because it offered one of the best biomedical engineering educations in the country, both were top students in the department, and both planned to go on to graduate studies in medicine or biomedical engineering. I first met them in the spring of 2004 as they sprinted to the finish line of their senior projects.

Kudesia, whose parents were from India, spent his early years in Guyana before moving to Odessa, Texas, as a young boy. His mother died when he was 5, and his father—a physician and professor of medicine—dedicated his life to his sons, both of whom showed a strong scientific bent. Vick's father would bring home his medical textbooks for his sons to peruse, an experience that made an impression on the studious boys.

"I remember seeing a drawing of an arm with the skin on and then an arm with the skin off and the muscles and vessels underneath and saying, 'Hey, that's interesting, that's for me,'" recalled Kudesia.

He spent hours building elaborate structures out of Legos. When he was older, he disassembled an old computer to see how it worked. After taking advanced science and mathematics courses at Odessa High School in the ninth and tenth grades, he attended the Texas

Academy of Math and Sciences in Denton. A pivotal moment for Kudesia came when he visited a science museum with an exhibit that featured a pair of robotic legs on a unicycle. Students had to figure out in which order to push four buttons so that the robotic legs would peddle the cycle successfully—an exercise that fascinated Kudesia.

"I guess that's one of the things that first got me interested in combining the human body and engineering," said Kudesia.

Like many science-minded high school students, Kudesia at first had no idea that the discipline of biomedical engineering existed or that you could major in it in college. But a little Web surfing brought enlightenment on that score, and he applied to Boston University's Biomedical Engineering Department, entering the university in 2000. During his first two years he plowed through basic courses like chemistry, advanced calculus and physics, engineering mechanics, and principles of biology. But in his junior year he waded into the heart of BU's biomedical engineering curriculum, taking courses such as engineering physiology and biomechanics. Kudesia, like many other students, became hooked on the field when he took a course in control systems taught by Jim Collins, a popular young professor and recipient of both a Whitaker Foundation grant and a MacArthur fellowship, otherwise known as a "genius" award. In the course, Collins interweaves the principles that govern mechanical and electrical engineering with the far more intricate systems that control the human body. One of the first examples Collins gave his students was the elaborate system of controls and feedback that enables a person to walk normally, from the contact of feet to floor, to vision, to the inner ear's balance system.

"You were taught how to think about problems, how to get your arms around them, how to break a big problem down into its smaller components," said Kudesia, now in medical school at BU. "You were taught how to quantify the hell out of everything. . . . The human body is a complicated thing. All these systems are interlocking and talking back and forth. I want to get in there and use all these engineering principles to see what is happening and figure out the various parts."

Another important experience for Kudesia was working as a volunteer in the emergency room of the Boston City Hospital. There, despite all the medical advances in recent years, Kudesia saw the need for even more sophisticated devices, such as portable imaging machines that could rapidly scan a patient for internal injuries. "I saw these problems and I thought I could have the biggest impact if I went into medicine and took what I know from engineering and bridge these two worlds," he said.

With biomedical engineering professor John White as his adviser, Kudesia decided to investigate cardiac fibrillation. To model and compute how to halt fibrillation with a less powerful shock than is now used, he studied the many models of heart rhythm and fibrillation in the medical literature. The heart beats when an electrical current is transmitted from the top of the heart, at the sinus node, down through the rest of the heart in a spiral-like wave, causing the muscle to contract. A smoothly beating heart is a model of harmony and rhythm, but that order can be disrupted when heart muscle is damaged by a heart attack. Dead heart muscle does not properly transmit the heart's electrical signals, and as the electrical wave flows through the heart, it can sometimes get thrown out of whack as it hits the dead tissue, somewhat like a phonograph needle getting stuck on a record. In certain instances, this disorder feeds on itself, sending the heart into the turmoil of fibrillation.

Implantable defibrillators sense when the entire heart is beating erratically and administer a shock to jolt it back into its normal rhythm. Kudesia reasoned that since cardiac scar tissue is usually a hot spot of fibrillation, why not invent an electrode that could be placed squarely over the damaged portion of the heart and block the fibrillation as soon as it began, using a far less powerful current?

"Current devices wait until the problem has spread through all the heart and shock it full force," said Kudesia. "We hope to use less current and more finesse. It would be like going from a car battery to a double A battery."

Kudesia wrote hundreds of lines of computer code as he created a model of a heart beating in and out of sync. He experimented with different electrodes, rejecting a bull's-eye design and a parallel bar design before settling on his cross-shaped electrode. He ran into numerous obstacles, frequently consulting with postdoctoral student Tay Netoff when he hit a wall.

"In every other class you have homework and you know there's an answer to it," said Kudesia. "There's someone out there who knows how to do it already. In this project, I had help and I had papers I could read. But I had to connect all the dots into one functional piece. I suppose this is what you hope to learn in school, to link together these very different pieces of knowledge. It was like grabbing smoke and fashioning a form out of it. That's why this was so important to me. It was a test of whether I really grasped the fundamentals of all these classes. The classes were no longer isolated and abstract and I had to fashion together something that was functional. This has really given me confidence that I could do something like this."

Among Kudesia's more innovative ideas was to first administer a small negative charge to the heart—sort of like electrically clearing the decks—before zapping the cardiac tissue with a positive charge. His models showed that this set the stage for defibrillation and was more effective in yanking the heart back into rhythm. A few days before he was to present his project at the April conference, Kudesia rehearsed his presentation before White, Netoff, and nine graduate students. Although only a computer model, Kudesia's research and crisp delivery left the group impressed.

"It's easy to complete homework when you know there's an answer, but this was open-ended," said Netoff. "This was a six-month project that involved him breaking the problem down into steps he could achieve. He had to come up with novel solutions for problems he'd never encountered before. Vick showed great enthusiasm from the beginning. He just took the reins and ran with it."

Like Vick Kudesia, Inas Khayal was a teenager when she realized she wanted to invent new technologies to improve human health. Born in Palestine, Khayal moved to Saudi Arabia when she was a little girl, then immigrated to the United States with her family at age 12. The daughter of a dentist and an electrical engineer, Khayal excelled at math and science at her public high school in Abington,

Massachusetts, near Boston. In the summer after her junior year in high school, she and her older sister volunteered to work in a school for disabled children in the Gaza Strip. She was dismayed by the lack of tools and equipment and resolved to devote her education and career to advancing medicine.

"I was thinking of doing engineering or medicine in college," said Khayal, a striking woman with dark eyes and the poise of someone many years older. "But after my time in Gaza I was positive I wanted to do biomedical engineering. There was one girl there, about 5 years old, and she had severe disabilities in her knees. But the doctors couldn't do anything about it because there was such a lack of instrumentation and equipment. That's what really struck me. The doctors were there, but without the devices you couldn't do anything for these people. What is a doctor if he doesn't have the tools he needs? That's when I decided I wanted to bring these two things together."

During Khayal's freshman year at BU, her mother, then 48, was diagnosed with colon cancer, which only increased the young woman's desire to work in medicine. But like many biomedical engineering students, she realized she was more interested in inventing new devices and therapies than directly treating patients.

"I really wanted to do something that was going to benefit people," said Khayal. "I could be a doctor or engineer but feel I could be of more benefit as an engineer. I want to design things, but I also want to work closely with doctors to understand what people need. I want to make sure that the work I do gets applied and translated into devices that actually get used.... My overall philosophy about biomedical engineering is that if you can't see a product or a benefit for the patient in five or ten years, I'm not really inspired to work on it."

Her conviction to become a biomedical engineer was affirmed in her junior year when she took a physiology course. She found that while many of the premed students were interested in absorbing as much information as possible, she and her fellow biomedical engineering majors were more intrigued with why the body functioned the way it did. Her sentiment was expressed by many biomedical engineering students, who are often more interested in breaking down physiological systems into functions that can be quantified, modeled, and predicted.

"I enjoyed physiology, but I had lots of questions about why things worked, rather than just being told how they worked and to memorize it," said Khayal.

By her junior year, Khayal—who had summer internships at biomedical engineering companies such as GE Medical Systems and Boston Scientific Corporation—was increasingly interested in studying imaging. She began to work with Professor Bigio, a leading researcher in biomedical optics and photonics. These fields involve using different kinds of light to do everything from determining whether cells are cancerous to activating drugs inside the body.

For Khayal's senior project, Bigio put her to work on an investigation in which he has a keen interest and which could one day play a role in cancer diagnosis and treatment. When oncologists administer chemotherapy to cancer patients, their tumor cells die through a process of apoptosis, or programmed cell death. Sometimes it can take weeks before pathologists, using the conventional method of looking at slides under a microscope, can tell if a chemotherapy regime is working.

Bigio is convinced there is a better way. Normal cells and cells undergoing apoptosis have a different density, as well as variations in the DNA of their nuclei, and Bigio believes that by shining laser light on the cells you can tell the difference. Khayal's task was to develop an instrument that could measure the difference between normal cells and cells dying from chemotherapy, based on the directions in which light scatters as it refracts off the cells. The ultimate goal, said Bigio, is to get a tiny, fiber-optical probe close to a cancer treatment site—through either an endoscope or a fine needle—and tell immediately whether a cancer therapy is working. If not, oncologists could quickly switch to a new drug regimen.

"There is a loss of valuable time if treatment is not working, and you may need to switch to more aggressive care," said Bigio.

Despite her ample self-confidence, Khayal was initially daunted by the project. Constructing the laser device involved a considerable amount of electrical and mechanical engineering, fields in which she had limited experience. But with the help of postdoctoral fellow Ousama a'Amar, she built an instrument that illuminated a vial of cells with a laser beam. A detector then automatically rotated around the vial, moving 1.125 degrees every few seconds and taking about 10,000 measurements of the scattered light from every angle.

Two nights before her presentation, I found Khayal in Bigio's fifth-floor lab in the Photonics Building, working past midnight to hone her results. She turned off the lights in the lab, and when she set the instrument in motion, countless tiny red dots—the scattered laser light from the cells—whirled around on the walls. Her results were rough but seemed to follow a pattern: The apoptotic cells, whose irregular, disintegrating nuclei contained more smaller particles than regular cells, tended to scatter the laser light backward more than forward.

Her senior project presentation, the last of the day, went well. She noted that 500,000 Americans die every year from cancer, with 1.3 million new cases reported annually. Optical detection and monitoring may eventually prove to be a new weapon in the war on cancer, said Khayal, who, after graduation, entered a Ph.D. program in biomedical imaging run jointly by the University of California, San Francisco, Medical School and UC Berkeley. Chemotherapy-induced apoptosis usually occurs within two to three days, she said, adding, "If we're able to detect this earlier, that would be very valuable."

After the conference was over, BU's biomedical engineering faculty named Khayal's the most outstanding senior project.

Bigio said her work played an important role in showing his lab what still needed to be done to detect cell death using optics. These include a higher-quality laser and a better detector to measure the intensity of light scattering off the cells.

"It's a start," said Bigio. "But that's what's great about the senior project. We just don't invent a project for them. We look at what part of our research program we need to look farther into, and the kids sink their teeth into it and get a lot out of it. But we want to get something out of it, too. We want to do research that matters to our program.

"Inas started gradually with this project, but she really turned on the afterburners in the last two months. I think these senior projects are a crucial element in the undergraduate experience here. It's a much more intense effort than they've ever experienced, and it gets them closer to the scientific community. They graduate as full-fledged biomedical engineers, which they wouldn't have been without this project."

Inas Khayal, Vick Kudesia, and their classmates in Boston University's Biomedical Engineering Department personify a new breed of student steeped in a cross-disciplinary blend of engineering, biology, and medicine. This new field has been defined in many ways, but all come down to roughly the same thing: applying the science of engineering—with its mathematical equations, computer modeling, and aim of understanding the fundamental workings of physical systems—to medicine.

"For years the prevailing view was that physicians were largely intuitive, artful practitioners," said William R. Brody, an M.D.-Ph.D. who is the president of the Johns Hopkins University. "Now you want to bring sophisticated engineering techniques to bear on major medical problems."

Michael Lysaght of Brown University defines biomedical engineering as "the application of engineering skills and disciplines to living systems." BU's Ken Lutchen has a slightly more elaborate explanation of what constitutes this emerging field: "BME is the integration and synthesis of engineering, mathematics, physics and computer science with biological systems to understand how biological systems work and use that understanding to improve health care and treat disease."

One thing on which everyone can agree is the rapidly growing popularity of biomedical engineering as an undergraduate major and its ability to attract large numbers of female students into engineering, the traditional domain of men. More than 40 percent of biomedical engineering students in American universities are women, double the percentage in classic engineering disciplines, such as civil and mechanical engineering. The reason, most biomedical engineers agree, is that women are drawn to a field that has a direct impact on saving lives and improving health care.

"I liked the fact that you could actually develop things that could help people," said Tejal Desai, a Boston University associate professor of biomedical engineering and one of the young female stars in the field. "It was the inventing and thinking I could make a singular impact with something I created."

In this era of the biological revolution, it's also not surprising that many engineers would turn away from designing turbines or aircraft and focus instead on understanding the human body and disease—down to the genetic and molecular level—using engineering systems. And given the explosion of information in biology and genetics, it's crucial that engineers working in medicine receive the broad education offered at major universities.

"There is so much technology out there that you have to have individuals trained in technology and biomedicine to make a big impact," said Michael Berns, a founder of the Beckman Laser Center and the Biomedical Engineering Center at the University of California, Irvine. "Fifty or one hundred years ago there were medical technologies, but you could count them on one hand at any given time. Now the technologies are so much more numerous and complex. The evolution of bioengineering in the last thirty years came about as a necessity. People now have to be trained in multiple disciplines in order to solve pieces of the puzzle. The sheer volume and complexity of the technologies have mandated that you have to train people in a new way and in multiple disciplines."

In recent years, the inexorable march of biology and medicine down to the molecular and genetic level has brought about a fundamental shift in biomedical engineering. For several decades, the field was ruled by the men and women who made devices: pacemakers, left ventricular heart pumps, kidney dialysis machines, artificial hips, imaging machines. Inevitably, however, the field is moving from the device level to the cellular level. One day, cardiac devices may be replaced by genetic engineering techniques that can repair damaged heart tissue. Artificial hips may fall out of favor as biomedical engineers and orthopedic researchers figure out how to combat diseases such as rheumatoid arthritis using molecular and cellular therapies.

No one is predicting the end of the devices that have defined biomedical engineering to date, only that they will increasingly share the stage with a new kind of biomedical engineering, one you can't touch or see with the human eye. Dan Hammer, chairman of the Department of Biomedical Engineering at the University of Pennsylvania, put it this way:

"For biomedical engineering to be successful it will have to blend the old device orientation and quantitative cell biology. We as engineers have certain tool sets that biologists don't necessarily have, and we're trying to discover some fundamental things: How do cell systems work? Can I engineer or manipulate that cell for treatment?"

Boston University's department epitomizes the blend of the old and the new, with numerous laboratories doing research in such diverse areas as tissue engineering, brain and vision research, biomedical optics, nanotechnology, cellular and subcellular mechanics, lung function, and genomics. In Jim Collins's Applied Biodynamics Laboratory, biomedical engineering research is taking place at all levels. On the genetic level, he and a team of graduate students and postdoctoral fellows are attempting to figure out what genes, or combination of genes, turn on the proteins that drive physiology and disease.

"Think of it being like the electrical wiring in your house, except in this case we have no wiring diagram," said Collins, who is 39. "So we're in the basement and we're trying to figure out which combination of switches will turn power on and off in different rooms of the house. That's effectively what we're doing. We're trying to figure out how these genes are wired up, who are the key guys, which ones should you knock out or turn off."

On the other end of the spectrum is Attila Priplata. A Ph.D. student in Collins's lab, Priplata is a traditional biomedical engineer, a device guy intent upon seeing his inventions brought into clinical use in fairly short order. Building on earlier research done by Collins, he has developed a device that may help the elderly and infirm maintain their balance and avoid falls.

About 33 percent of people over 65 years old fall every year. And about a third of these falls are due to a simple physiological fact: as people age, or experience nerve damage caused by diabetes, they can't feel the ground the way they once did. One way to help them is to increase their sensory perception of the ground, and Collins and Priplata have done this by inventing a pair of thin soles that emit vibrations just below the level that patients can feel. This subsensory "noise," as Priplata calls it, is fed to the patient's brain and significantly improves his or her balance. Priplata has tested this by attaching reflective markers to the patients and using a camera to precisely measure how much they sway front to back and side to side, with and without the vibrating soles. With the soles, the postural sway of many elderly can be reduced to the point where they wobble no more than young, healthy experimental subjects. Priplata believes the soles will also help improve the balance of people with Parkinson's disease, multiple sclerosis, and neurological damage from strokes.

"As a way of measuring and quantifying the body, biomedical engineering was very appealing to me," said Priplata, who is working with a company to manufacture the vibrating soles. "Genetics just didn't appeal to me. It's too micro. I wanted something I could see. I wanted to be able to interact with the human body on the organ level. I love the device side of biomedical engineering, and there's a lot to be done in the area of motor control. This is classical biomedical engineering. It's fortunate that I love it. But unfortunately we're a dying breed. Biomedical engineering is moving toward the cellular and subcellular side."

There is some truth in Priplata's lament, although ample room remains for working with devices in biomedical engineering. Indeed, Tejal Desai's laboratory is experimenting with technologies that combine devices with cellular biomedical engineering. Desai is BU's resident expert on micro-electrical-mechanical systems—MEMS, for short—which employ small devices to mimic organ function or deliver drugs. She has patented a MEMS device—containing pancreatic islet cells—that may one day be implanted in diabetics and assume the function of diseased pancreases.

Boston University's sweeping approach to a biomedical engineering education is typical of the best programs in the country. But what sets BU apart is its senior project, which its graduates remember as part boot camp, part transforming experience. Ken Lutchen—a hyperkinetic, plainspoken, 49-year-old New Yorker—is the driving force behind the project and a man who has played a key role in BU's rise to the top ranks of biomedical engineering.

When Lutchen first came to BU in 1985, the department had seven faculty members and a few thousand feet of lab space. Today, it has five times as many faculty and 45,000 square feet of lab space. The first senior project conference attracted representatives from seven companies. In 2004, fifty biomedical engineering firms sent observers to the conference. Today, 40 percent of BU's biomedical engineering seniors go on to graduate school, and 10 to 15 percent head to medical school. The rest go into industry, where the demand for biomedical engineers has soared since the mid-1980s.

Every year, Lutchen teaches a course instructing the seniors how to handle their senior project and prepare for life in the real world. He teaches them how to write résumés, prepare papers, and give oral presentations. I sat in on one class in November, during which he gave two presentations to the students—one a first-rate scientific paper, the other an obtuse talk with unintelligible slides. He was painting the students a stark picture of victory and defeat.

"You are actually creating a potential project from nothing," Lutchen told the students in the modern, U-shaped classroom with desks arrayed in several tiers. "This will be judged by your peers, faculty, and senior people in industry who will ask, 'Does this person really know what he's talking about?' Your oral presentation is an extraordinarily important and powerful skill set, and it is so hard to do well. To do this in ten minutes is very hard. But it's unbelievably important. It's a very efficient way for you to convince a lot of people of what you have accomplished. It's also a very efficient way for you to destroy what people think of you as a competent bioengineer. Are these people going to say that this guy doesn't have a clue what he's talking about?"

I sat in on another senior project class in early April, a few weeks before the project conference. The students had begun their final push to complete their papers, and many looked weary. Lutchen was all exhortation.

"You should be going at it 125 percent!" he said. "This is your chance. If you drop the ball now, you've really lost an opportunity. It's three more weeks and it's over. So go crazy! Get a little less sleep."

Just a few days before the conference, Lutchen listened to the seniors in his pulmonary function lab run through the first of two dress rehearsals. He was restless, frequently interjecting comments and criticisms. When one young woman flashed a series of lung CT scans rapidly onto the screen, Lutchen interjected, "This is really cool stuff. Don't be in a rush to get through it. This is not torture."

Another young woman started her rambling talk by showing a couple of indecipherable slides, causing Lutchen to practically leap out of his chair.

"Get this off!" he told her. "This is garbage. . . . Back up! Back up! Back up! Where are you going?"

Sitting in his office after the first rehearsal, he told me, "This always happens. The first dry run is a disaster."

Lutchen believed in keeping the heat on until the end, convinced it was better for him to ruthlessly dissect his students' talks rather than let them flop at the conference. His approach to the project—and, indeed, to his students' entire education—was almost messianic.

"It goes without saying that you've got to give students the basic, fundamental knowledge," Lutchen said. "But what distinguishes the best programs are those that teach lifelong learning skills. This project teaches them to be individually accountable for the quality of their work. It teaches them how to be resourceful. It teaches them how to work on large, complex projects in the lab. Most importantly, it teaches them that they can take on a very substantive challenge and succeed at a very high level. No experience prepares them to deal with the challenges of the real world as much as this."

Chapter 3

Beyond the Artificial Heart

Roxanne Emswiler was the sort of person who almost never got sick. She only occasionally caught a cold, rarely had the flu. Other than when giving birth to her two children, she had managed to avoid hospitals. So it came as something of a shock when, in 2000, at age 47, she came down with a terrible, early-spring cold. Within a day she felt miserable. And by the second or third day she felt so lousy and was so out of breath that the trim, fit bank teller was admitted to Rockingham Memorial Hospital in her hometown of Harrisonburg, Virginia.

Soon, it was clear that Emswiler had more than a cold. A series of tests revealed that her heart was pumping at less than a quarter of its normal capacity, its rate had jumped to twice normal speed, and so much fluid was accumulating around her heart and in her lungs that she could scarcely draw a breath. Alarmed at her deteriorating condition, her physician in Harrisonburg—suspecting heart failure—transferred her to the University of Virginia Hospital in Charlottesville, a top cardiac center. There, doctors quickly made a diagnosis: Emswiler had myocarditis, a type of heart failure that wreaks havoc with the organ's ability to contract. Hers was the most frightening form, one in which a virus suddenly attacks the heart muscle of a healthy person and, within days or weeks, destroys its ability to function.

Dr. James D. Bergin, the director of the University of Virginia's Heart Failure and Transplantation Program, knew the situation was desperate. He placed Emswiler on the heart transplant list. But to keep her alive in the meantime, Bergin knew she would need a device that, in recent years, had saved the lives of thousands of people like Emswiler. It was a classic piece of biomedical engineering, known as a left ventricular assist device, or LVAD. More than twice the size of a hockey puck and weighing 2½ pounds, the LVAD would replace Emswiler's left ventricle, or chamber, which performs 80 percent of the heart's labor as it squeezes oxygenated blood through the aorta to the rest of the body.

Bergin called in Dr. Curt Tribble, U. Va.'s top cardiac surgeon, who concurred that Emswiler needed an LVAD if she was to survive long enough for a transplant. The operation was scheduled for the same week, but by the time Tribble implanted the LVAD, Emswiler was so close to death that Bergin feared she would expire on the way from her fourth-floor room to the second-floor operating suite.

In an operation lasting five hours, Tribble opened up Emswiler, stopped her heart, placed her on a heart-lung bypass machine, and sewed the LVAD's synthetic vessels to the vessels of Emswiler's rapidly deteriorating left ventricle. He connected the synthetic vessels to the LVAD, which rested in her abdominal cavity just below her diaphragm. Tribble then cut a hole through her abdominal wall and pulled and tugged an electrical line—which would power the LVAD—through the opening. Taking Emswiler off the heart-lung bypass machine, Tribble restarted her heart by filling it with blood; he then turned on the VLAD, which rocked powerfully inside her. The machine, known as the HeartMate and invented by engineer Victor L. Poirier, assumed the function of the left ventricle while working in concert with the rest of Emswiler's heart.

The operation was, in effect, an elaborate plumbing procedure inside the human body. As Tribble, a handsome, lanky 52-year-old, told me after I observed a different LVAD operation, "I learned more about heart surgery and VADs working on my car in my parents' barn than I ever learned in a formal environment."

When the operation was over, Emswiler was alive and tethered to a portable machine the size of a large briefcase. As she began the wait for a new heart, teams of engineers, including some at the University of Virginia, were working to create new ventricular assist devices that were the stuff of dreams for surgeons such as Tribble: devices as small as a person's thumb and totally contained within the body.

The LVAD is a remarkable device, yet despite everything these pumps are doing—and promise to do—for patients, their development does not represent the frontier of cardiovascular biomedical engineering. Crudely put, the LVAD is twentieth-century technology. The twenty-first century is likely to be dominated not by machines that replace already broken hearts but by bioengineering advances at the cellular and genetic level that will thwart the very processes that cause heart disease in the first place. Like almost every field of biomedical engineering, heart research is moving beyond the devices that have helped millions of patients—cardiac pacemakers, implantable defibrillators, arterial stents, mechanical pumps—to a new world of engineering the genes, proteins, and cells that are the building blocks of the human body.

To get a sense of where cardiovascular research is heading in this new century, you need only walk a long block from the operating room where Roxanne Emswiler received an LVAD. In a recently constructed brick-and-glass building at the heart of the University of Virginia's rapidly expanding medical research complex are the labs of the Department of Biomedical Engineering and the Cardiovascular Research Center. There, scores of researchers—some biomedical engineers, some physicians, some molecular biologists—are investigating the fundamental processes that lead to diseases of the heart and blood vessels. The importance of such work is underscored by a simple fact: of the roughly 2.5 million Americans who die every year, 37 percent—about 950,000 people—succumb to cardiovascular disease.

Employing a broad array of engineering tools—superpowerful computers, experimental imaging techniques, devices that enable scientists to photograph moving blood cells—the researchers are tackling several basic challenges. One is unraveling the process of how white blood cells and fatty cells penetrate arterial walls and form the plaques that expand, burst, and block arteries, cutting off blood supply and causing a heart attack. University of Virginia investigators are trying to learn more about the molecular signaling that takes place at the start of that cascade, a complex dance in which the cells lining artery walls send out messages that attract white blood cells, which then slow down, stop, and set in motion the inflammation that plays a key role in plaque formation. The ultimate goal is to help develop a drug, and possibly a genetic therapy, that will nip vessel inflammation and plaque accretion in the bud.

Other researchers are working to decipher the genetic and cellular mysteries underlying the heart failure that often follows a heart attack. Even if only a small portion of cardiac muscle is damaged in a heart attack, that dead zone can wreak havoc with the heart's electrical rhythms. Molecules that inflame and ultimately weaken cardiac cells are also released by the remaining healthy heart tissue. This destructive process, which is the body's way of compensating for the damage caused by a heart attack, is known as cardiac "remodeling" and can lead to congestive heart failure. A group of U. Va. biomedical engineers is studying heart remodeling in mice by tying off a coronary artery, inducing a heart attack, and then using advanced imaging techniques and chemical tests to monitor the heart as it weakens, stretches, and loses its ability to pump. Their goal is to discover better ways to prevent heart remodeling, including genetically reprogramming heart muscle to make it resistant to remodeling. Physicians now treat remodeling with some success using various drugs.

Thomas C. Skalak, the 47-year-old chairman of U. Va.'s Department of Biomedical Engineering, sees all this work heading in one direction: to an understanding of the cardiovascular system from the genetic level all the way to the miraculous synchrony of the beating heart and using that knowledge to prevent disease. It is a lofty goal, one that may not be attained in Skalak's lifetime. But like many biomedical engineers, Skalak believes it is possible to break down the cardiovascular system into its component parts and then, using massive computing power and the rapidly unfolding secrets of genetics, put it all together to prevent and treat disease. He likens the process to assembling a very intricate watch. Right now, biomedical engineers and other researchers have the innards of the watch spread out before them. The challenge is to figure out how all the pieces fit together—a task perfectly suited to engineers, Skalak contends.

"Biology is a network of complex systems and engineers are good at complex systems," said Skalak, whose department has nearly doubled in size recently, to 18 full-time faculty, 80 graduate students, and 180 undergraduates. "Now with the sequencing of the genome, we are beginning to know all the building blocks. The question is, how do they fit together? If I hand you all the parts of a watch, could you make the watch work? That's what the field we now call digital biology or systems biology is about, learning how it all goes together to make a functioning system. It's like the difference between a metallurgist and a watchmaker. A metallurgist knows all the materials that go into making a watch. But only the watchmaker knows how to put it all together."

Putting it all together will enable doctors to practice what Skalak and others call reparative or regenerative medicine—using engineering to help the body prevent and fight disease.

"Bioengineering is not the six million dollar man," said Skalak. "It's harnessing what from an evolutionary point of view is the most amazing creation of nature. We have to understand human biological systems well enough so we see how they work and how we can manipulate them. Preventative or reparative medicine is where the future of biomedical engineering is. My vision is that we get good enough at biomedical engineering that we can do much more preventative medicine. You'll know what's going on early through imaging. Is an organ having a problem? If so, we will give appropriate mechanical or drug intervention so we can instruct the body's reparative system to go into action."

Understanding the complex mechanisms behind the deposition of plaque in arteries and using drugs or genetic engineering to prevent or treat it is only one example of reparative medicine. Another is the LVAD itself. In patients stricken with virus-induced cardiac disease, the heart can sometimes recover much of its function after the virus has run its course. Not only does the LVAD keep patients alive when the heart is unable to pump enough blood, but studies show that the strong, regular beating of the LVAD-assisted heart can actually help weakened heart cells recover, enabling some patients to be weaned off the pump.

No biomedical engineers, including Skalak, say that the unraveling of the secrets of genes and cells will eliminate the need for devices like the LVAD. After a burst of sometimes euphoric and overly optimistic predictions in the 1990s—with some saying that hearts and other organs would be grown in labs in a decade or two—biomedical engineers are more realistic these days. The universe of the genome is vast and intricate, with complex combinations of genes and proteins responsible for even the most basic functions of the cardiovascular system. Such complexity can daunt investigators, but Skalak advocates a slow, steady approach, believing that researchers should bite off realistic challenges and be mindful of how their work can be translated into patient benefit.

"You don't want to stop the forward march of medicine because you don't understand everything," said Skalak.

With America facing an aging baby boom population and an epidemic of obesity, cardiologists are going to need all the help they can get from biomedical engineers. That became evident when I spent an afternoon in the University of Virginia's cardiac clinic shadowing Jonathan R. Lindner, a cardiologist and associate professor of medicine at the university. A trim, energetic, quick-witted man who looks younger than his 40 years, Lindner not only sees patients but also works closely with the university's biomedical engineers on several research projects. During the hours I was at Lindner's side, I gained an appreciation for the toll that smoking, overeating, and lack of exercise are taking on the country's collective cardiovascular health. Indeed, to spend a day in the cardiac clinic of a major university medical center is to come away amazed that, despite the harm people inflict on themselves, the nation's life expectancy continues to climb and that deaths from cardiovascular disease have even dropped slightly in the past several years. This is a testament to the advances in biomedical engineering and surgery—think pacemakers and heart bypass operations—as well as to the development of cardiac wonder drugs, such as beta-blockers, which settle the heart's rhythm, and statins, which lower cholesterol. To some degree, these cheering statistics are also due to the dedication of some Americans—still a minority—who adopt healthier lifestyles.

Among Lindner's patients was a 58-year-old man who stood 5 feet, 9 inches tall and weighed 252 pounds. He had a litany of ailments common to the obese: diabetes, high blood pressure, sleep apnea, congestive heart failure. A former smoker, he had a leaky heart valve and had had several heart attacks. He had severe atherosclerosis—arteries impeded by deposits of fat and plaque—and surgeons had performed a balloon angioplasty to reopen some of those vessels. To treat his apnea, he slept with a mask that forced air down his throat. No doubt he had brought many of these afflictions upon himself, but he also was probably saddled with bad cholesterol genes that worsened his coronary artery disease. The man had been a longtime patient of Lindner's, and at Lindner's urging he had begun to diet—losing 15 pounds—and had started to exercise. Lindner restarted a drug that the man's local physician in North Carolina had discontinued and wrote the man half a dozen prescriptions.

Following this man was another male patient, aged 60, who would clinically be described as morbidly obese. Standing 6 feet tall and weighing 325 pounds, the man carried around a belly nearly the size of a beer keg. He had smoked until 1991, when, experiencing chest pains, he went in for tests and wound up having quadruple coronary artery bypass surgery. The arteries in his legs were being steadily narrowed by plaque, which caused him pain in his lower extremities. He, too, was diabetic. The man, a relatively new patient of Lindner's, asked about losing weight and getting some exercise. After examining him, Lindner told the patient about a university clinic that treats overweight people who have both heart disease and diabetes. The patient vowed to sign up.

I was impressed by how much time Lindner spent with this man and other patients—many were with him for up to half an hour—and told him so. Lindner, dressed in khaki pants, a light green shirt, and tie, replied, "I spent a little more time with him than I do with most people. But at least I showed I care and he knows I care and perhaps he'll care a little more himself."

To win the war against heart disease, biomedical engineers at the University of Virginia are not counting on a sudden turnaround in the eating habits and lifestyles of most Americans. They place more faith in their own ability to discover new ways to drastically slow the processes that lead to heart attacks and strokes. As Brent A. French, a leading researcher of heart remodeling, put it, "Cardiovascular disease is eminently preventable. And that's what makes it all the more tragic because people do it to themselves. The rural Japanese before World War II had extremely low cholesterol levels and very little heart disease. But after the war many of them adopted a more American diet and they started dropping like flies. It's sad. And it's equally sad that people take pills more readily than they take advice."

Trained as a biochemist and molecular biologist, French initially did research in medical schools at the Baylor College of Medicine and the University of Louisville. Deciding he wanted to tackle heart disease in a more direct, interdisciplinary way, he joined the University of Virginia's Biomedical Engineering Department in 1998. Today, he and his team are working on one of the great challenges in cardiovascular medicine: Why do patients' hearts remodel and weaken after heart attacks, and how can that degenerative process be thwarted? His knowledge of molecular biology and genetics is vital to this enterprise, but so, too, are the tools of biomedical engineering, such as employing magnetic resonance imaging.

"Biomedical engineering offers a strategic location where you can combine the elements of engineering, medicine, and molecular biology," said French, a courtly, mustachioed associate professor who speaks in a soft, southern accent. "Ultimately it is the interface of all these disciplines that appealed to me. It provides me with an opportunity to do what I couldn't have done otherwise. Biomedical engineering lets me get extremely close to medicine while still maintaining connections to the basic sciences and engineering."

Another aspect—rooted, no doubt, in the field's early dominance by practical-minded engineers and inventors—also appeals to French: the striving to bring therapies to patients as quickly as possible.

"In biomedical engineering there is total acceptance of focusing on a disease and saying, 'Okay, we are just going to go all out and find ways to optimize the diagnosis and treatment of this particular disease,'" French said. "You lay everything on the table and you say, 'We are taking all of the tools available to us from these diverse fields and we are going to make an all-out assault on this disease.' That's not always accepted in basic science departments, where sometimes there is an almost aloof attitude that if your research is too applied it's no longer good science. But there is no such thing as being too applied in biomedical engineering. . . . I think most of us have this basic motivation to do something worthwhile with our lives and benefit mankind. That's my fundamental motivation. Maybe biomedical engineers are a bunch of frustrated physicians. We may not lay our hands on the patient, but we can certainly invent tools to put into the doctors' hands."

To better understand heart remodeling, French's team is working with genetically engineered mice whose heart muscle lacks a gene that appears to play a major role in the debilitating process. This gene controls the production of an enzyme called iNOS—short for inducible nitric oxide synthase—that can alter the way heart muscle contracts. After a heart attack, the inflammatory iNOS enzyme hinders the heart's ability to contract, particularly in the crucial left ventricle. That phenomenon, coupled with the poor way in which damaged heart muscle conducts electrical currents, means that some heart attack survivors, if not placed on medication, may experience such severe remodeling that they die of congestive heart failure or sudden cardiac death within six to nine months. Even those placed on medication can experience remodeling and weakening of their heart in the months following a large myocardial infarction. In mice, as well as humans, the heart tries to make up for its lost pumping ability by growing larger, which has the effect of thinning out the heart's walls and making it pump even less efficiently.

"This is a global dysfunction brought about by the local dysfunction produced by a heart attack," said French.

He and his co-workers have done groundbreaking work showing that mice lacking the gene for the pro-inflammatory iNOS enzyme do not experience the same cardiac remodeling after a heart attack. Mice in which a gene has been removed—known as "knockout" mice—are produced by isolating a particular gene, making a mutant version of the gene that neutralizes its function, and then introducing that mutant gene into embryonic mouse stem cells. Those cells are then used to produce mice that lack, for example, the iNOS gene, meaning that the information necessary to produce the enzyme has literally been "knocked out" of their genetic repertoire. The use of knockout, or genetically engineered, mice has become a vital tool in research laboratories worldwide. So far, investigators have identified and "knocked out" about 3,000 of the more than 20,000 genes found in mice.

French has induced heart attacks in normal, or "wild type," mice and in iNOS knockout mice and then followed their progress over the course of twenty-eight days. The results have been striking. After a month, the heart of the regular mouse, which still has the inflammatory iNOS gene, has grown significantly, its thinning walls able to pump only a small fraction of blood out of the heart. "Under repeated pressure the dead tissue bulges and expands," said French. "The heart tried to maintain its spherical shape and the undamaged tissue thins out."

But the heart of the knockout mouse, lacking the iNOS gene, still functions fairly well, although the muscle tissue damaged by the heart attack still does not contract properly. At twenty-eight days after the heart attack, the hearts of the knockout mice are generally half the size of the normal mice hearts that underwent remodeling.

"If you take out the iNOS gene, you effectively block left ventricular remodeling," said French. "The bottom line is we've almost completely prevented the heart remodeling process. We've knocked it out with a knockout mouse. We've proven genetically that iNOS is a bad player in the progression of heart failure."

The ultimate goal of such research is to figure out a way to block left ventricular remodeling in the heart, perhaps with drugs, perhaps by turning certain genes on or off. "We're examining ways to genetically reprogram heart muscle to make it resistant to disease," said French. "We want to offer protection against heart failure after a heart attack. . . . The Centers for Disease Control is predicting an epidemic of heart disease, because by the year 2010 there will be 40 million Americans over 65. More people are surviving heart attacks because of better medical care and many will have a lot of damaged heart tissue. And if large portions of the heart sustain damage, it's almost like a death sentence. A large heart attack is like tipping over a stack of dominoes. The bigger the infarction, the more the heart expands, and the more the heart expands, the more likely you are to suffer heart failure and death."

The manipulation of genes to fight disease is exceedingly complex, not least because destructive processes such as heart remodeling are likely the result of an array of genes kicking into gear and altering numerous proteins that control human physiology. The safety of doing such genetic engineering in humans also is unproven. For these reasons, many leading investigators think that practical genetic therapies for cardiovascular disease are perhaps a decade away from use in humans. For the short term at least, drug therapies are more promising, and U. Va. researcher Joel Linden has discovered a drug, called ATL146e, that has promising anti-inflammatory effects on cardiac tissue.

A key member of French's heart research team is Dr. Zequan Yang, an assistant professor of biomedical engineering and a former heart surgeon in Beijing. By tying off the coronary arteries of mice, he induces heart attacks in the creatures. Once he does so, in both normal and genetically engineered mice, other researchers use advanced MRI, computer processing, and biochemical tests to study the remodeling process.

Mice, widely used in biomedical engineering experiments, have hearts that beat about 600 times per minute—about 10 times as rapidly as a human heart. This fast rate may be related to the speed with which their hearts remodel, making mice well suited to cardiac studies. After inducing a heart attack in the mice, Yang studies the effect on heart remodeling over the course of a month. After overdosing the animals with anesthesia, he removes the hearts, sections them, and then freezes them for later study of the physiological changes brought about by oxygen-depriving heart attacks.

French and his fellow U. Va. investigators have obtained what may be the best magnetic resonance (MR) images in the world of mouse hearts after an infarct. Once the images have been produced, Frederick H. Epstein, an associate professor of radiology and biomedical engineering, subjects them to a computer program he has devised, one that divides the heart into hundreds of sectors. The computer then crunches the data from those sectors to come up with a three-dimensional picture showing precisely which parts of the heart are contracting properly and which are debilitated.

One afternoon, French and Epstein sat in a control room in a medical research building, just a few feet from an adjoining room that contained an experimental MRI machine—about 5 feet square—three times as powerful as conventional MRI machines. Inside this contraption was a mouse whose cells were being subjected to a magnetic force 90,000 times more powerful than the earth's magnetic field. Such power causes the protons inside different types of cells to snap to magnetic attention in different ways and then return to their normal position when the MRI pulse is turned off. This process provides a clear picture of tissues, bone, and blood and is excellent for imaging the heart. French and Epstein were looking at black-and-white images of a mouse heart beating on a computer screen. They pointed out the thinning and bulging of the left ventricular wall, as well as blood pooling in the heart—all signs that this was a "wild type" mouse whose heart had remodeled after a heart attack.

Epstein said that such accurate MR images, coupled with computer programs that can minutely analyze cardiac muscle function, would give physicians a superb, noninvasive way of judging the condition of a patient's heart. But such advanced imaging and computer mapping is at least three to five years from coming to market, Epstein believes, as the technology must be refined and simplified so that radiologists and medical technicians can use it effortlessly.

Other U. Va. biomedical engineers and doctors are working on ways to make MRI as accurate as conventional, invasive methods of measuring the extent of blockage in a patient's arteries. Right now, in a procedure known as angiography, doctors insert a catheter into a patient's vein, inject a contrast agent through the catheter, and use an X-ray to see how much of an artery is blocked by plaque. But researchers at the University of Virginia, other universities, and imaging companies are swiftly overcoming a major hurdle with cardiovascular MRIs—that the beating heart and pulsing arteries cause too much interference with the images. The biomedical engineers at U. Va. can currently judge the extent of blockage with about 80 percent accuracy. Their aim is to soon attain 95 percent accuracy, which would make MRI a realistic alternative to angiography.

Dr. Christopher M. Kramer, an associate professor of medicine and radiology, works closely with U. Va. biomedical engineers on the cardiovascular MRI project. He believes that within a decade or two the MRI will be the "gold standard" in cardiovascular imaging. One morning in June 2004, I sat with Kramer as he took MR images of a 53-year-old woman who had been smoking for thirty years and had leg pain caused by partially blocked femoral arteries, which run through the groin. The woman was participating in a five-year study, funded by the National Institutes of Health, to evaluate atherosclerosis in peripheral arteries. Some of the patients in the study were receiving statins, cholesterol-lowering drugs, and some weren't.

On this morning, Kramer was conducting a test ideally suited for MRI. Known as a perfusion test, it would measure how much blood flowed to the woman's leg muscles after she exercised. Kramer would inject the patient with a contrast agent containing the element gadolinium and then would ask her to repeatedly press down on a pedal with her foot as the MRI machine ran. With the gadolinium in the patient's arteries and veins, Kramer could see not only how well blood made it past her partially blocked arteries but also how quickly blood flowed into her muscles during exercise—another indicator of the severity of blockage in her vessels.

Lying inside the hulking MRI machine, the woman tired of pumping the pedal after a minute or two. Kramer then injected the gadolinium into her veins. It took three times longer for blood to flow into her leg muscles than in a healthy patient.

Sitting behind a computer screen in a control room next to the MRI machine, Kramer pointed out the significant plaque buildup in the patient's superficial femoral artery, a common site of atherosclerosis. The MRI machine generates images of slices of tissue, and Kramer examined plaque formations at various spots along her artery. Free-flowing blood looked black on the screen. The arterial walls, and the plaque accreting just beneath them, were white.

"Here is an area of a lot of disease—this cloudy white spot," said Kramer. "You can't even see blood flowing through it. Just pick a plaque. Now here's a nice big lumen [opening] but down here is a lot more plaque. And here. This is all plaque. . . . In a healthy patient, all you see is a nice, round black area of blood flow, so she has a lot of plaque. We'll put her on a statin drug and in one year we'll see what happens to the wall of the artery, to see if there is less plaque and more lumen."

The close collaboration of doctors and engineers on such imaging systems is emblematic of the interdisciplinary work taking place at America's major universities, a phenomenon due in large measure to the rise of biomedical engineering.

"Engineers have been involved in every major tangible advance you can think of—heart-lung machines, stents, pacemakers, defibrillators," Dr. Arthur "Tim" Garson, dean of the University of Virginia Medical School, told me in an interview. "It's hard to imagine any advance that biomedical engineering has not been involved in. And that's the old biomedical engineering. Now the new biomedical engineering is much more involved in investigating basic biological systems. Biomedical engineering is a full partner at the table with the medical school. It's the closest ally we have at the University of Virginia."

Garson said that engineering-driven innovations in imaging, diagnosis, and treatment had made the practice of medicine much more of a science.

"At the patient's bedside thirty years ago, you used to be able to get by with, 'It's my opinion,' 'I wonder,' 'I think,' 'I guess,'" said Garson. "Now it's, 'Show me the data.' Now there's no more guessing involved."

Chapter 4

The Pump and Its Pipes

The research taking place at the University of Virginia's Biomedical Engineering Department is a testament to how far cardiovascular medicine has progressed in the past half century. Just before I was born, in 1952, physicians treated my ailing grandfather, who had high blood pressure and atherosclerosis, by placing him on a rice and honey diet. He died at age 51 of a massive stroke. Such was the woefully meager assortment of tools in physicians' and surgeons' bags in the mid-twentieth century, an era in which there were no cardiac pacemakers, no defibrillators, no arterial stents, no ventricular assist devices, no coronary artery bypass operations, very few effective cardiac drugs, and only the crudest of open-heart surgeries. If you had a serious cardiovascular condition in 1950, your prospects were only marginally better than they would have been in 1650.

All that began to change rapidly in the 1950s and 1960s, when an explosion in technology—driven, in part, by the invention of the transistor and the computer—led to a succession of inventions that dramatically increased the survival of people with ailing hearts. A crucial advance was the invention of the machine that took over the functions of the heart and lungs in the operating room, ushering in the era of open-heart surgery. The inventor was Philadelphia surgeon John Gibbon, who first used the machine on a patient in 1953 after twenty years of experimentation, sometimes using stray cats.

In 1957, Minnesota cardiac surgeon C. Walton Lillehei used the first externally powered pacemaker to treat a heart arrhythmia in a child. In 1958, Swedish surgeons placed the first implantable pacemaker in a patient. Two years later, an electrical engineer from Buffalo, New York, Wilson Greatbatch, employed two silicon transistors to create the first implantable pacemaker in the United States. Minnesota engineer Earl Bakken, working with Lillehei, played an important role in developing the first battery-powered pacemakers. Bakken formed a company, Medtronic, that is now the world's largest biomedical engineering firm, with annual sales of $9 billion and a workforce of 32,000 people worldwide.

In 1966, Houston heart surgeon Michael E. DeBakey implanted the first left ventricular assist device in a patient. The pump supported a woman for sixteen days until her own heart could fully resume pumping after valve repair surgery. In 1967, South African heart surgeon Christiaan Barnard performed the first human heart transplant. The patient lived eighteen days. That same year, the first coronary artery bypass surgery was performed at the Cleveland Clinic. In 1977, a Swiss physician performed the first angioplasty, giving birth to a procedure in which arterial plaque buildups are compressed using a balloon-like device inserted through a vessel in the groin. In 1982, the first artificial human heart—designed by Dr. Robert K. Jarvik—was implanted in patient Barney Clark. He lived 112 days. In 1987, doctors implanted the first arterial stents—scaffold-like devices that help keep arteries open after angioplasty.

Today, most of these procedures have become routine, helping prolong the lives of millions of people who might otherwise have had heart attacks, strokes, heart failure, or fatal cardiac arrhythmias. More than 2 million people worldwide now have cardiac pacemakers, with cardiologists implanting about 175,000 pacemakers annually in the United States. Doctors perform 2 million angioplasty procedures annually around the world, including 550,000 in America. Cardiologists in the United States perform about 500,000 coronary artery bypass operations a year and implant 800,000 stents.

But as the case of Emswiler's HeartMate pump shows, developing one of these lifesaving devices and bringing it to market can be a marathon journey. No one knows that better than Victor L. Poirier, the inventor of the HeartMate, the most widely used left ventricular assist device: it took twenty years and $62 million to develop the HeartMate and win approval from the U.S. Food and Drug Administration (FDA).

In the late 1960s, when Poirier first began work on the project at the request of the federal government, a sizable number of engineers and surgeons dreamed of creating a total artificial heart. But Poirier and his team of engineers at Thermo Cardiosystems Inc. soon deduced that creating an entire heart, with four separate chambers, would be a massive undertaking. Like good engineers, they broke the task into manageable pieces. Knowing that the left ventricle was the workhorse of the heart, they decided to create a device that would take over the functions of that chamber.

"When we first took a look at it we thought it would be a simple engineering problem," Poirier, a mechanical engineer, recalled. "Fundamentally the heart is just a pump and we were engineers and we figured we could deal with it. But we learned the hard way that that was not the case at all."

The challenges were enormous. The device had to be durable enough to beat 40 million times a year for at least two to three years. It had to be nontoxic and made of materials that could survive the corrosive saline environment of the human body. It had to pump blood at a velocity and volume roughly similar to those of a normal heart, which averages between 6 and 10 liters per minute. It had to pump blood without damaging delicate red blood cells. It had to have an ample supply of power and, perhaps most critical, had to sit in the body and do its work without causing blood clots, which could be fatal.

Poirier and his team of engineers came up with a basic design that would use pneumatic pressure from an external pump to drive a piston and diaphragm to pump blood. After eight years of testing 214 bladders and diaphragms, they discovered a type of polyurethane that could withstand being flexed tens of millions of times a year. After experimenting with pump bodies made of stainless steel, nickel, and other metals, Poirier settled on titanium as the ideal material because it did not react to the harsh environment inside the body and was quickly encased in a sack of scar tissue.

Then Poirier and his team turned to the toughest issue of all: finding a material that would not clot when it came in contact with the blood coursing through the pump. The engineers' initial instinct was to make diaphragms and vessels with a smooth surface, which, in combination with anticoagulant medicines, would prevent clotting. The results were disappointing. Then, in the early 1970s, Poirier and several engineers were sitting in a room in their Massachusetts laboratory, tossing ideas back and forth about nonclotting materials. Recently, pioneering heart surgeon Michael E. DeBakey had successfully invented vascular grafts made of woven material, which allowed cells to be deposited on the grafts and form a nonclotting natural surface. Why not, the engineers reasoned, coat surfaces of the pump with a similarly rough material?

"As engineers, we said the body naturally wants to form clots, so why don't we let it do that," recalled Poirier. "The whole concept was, 'Let's let it form clots but let's anchor them in place, hold them, so they can't be released into the bloodstream.'"

The result, still in use today, was a fibrous, porous surface that encouraged the deposition of the same endothelial cells that line human blood vessels—a design that has reduced the risk of complications from clotting to around 3 to 5 percent.

As Poirier continued his work in the early to mid-1970s, biomedical engineers and physicians at numerous universities also were developing different types of the ventricular assist device. One of the early pioneers was William Pierce of Pennsylvania State University, who in the 1970s invented a ventricular assist device to wean postoperative patients off a heart-lung machine.

By 1975, Poirier and his team of engineers had conducted extensive animal tests with the LVAD and were ready for human trials. Working with surgeons at the Texas Heart Institute, they devised a protocol in which LVADs would be implanted in twenty seriously ill patients whose hearts had been weakened after major cardiac surgery. The results were grim. The pump, which was then a cylindrical shape, as opposed to the current circular design, performed poorly.

Many of the patients perished within hours. One lived eight days. All would likely have died without the LVAD, but the results were nevertheless a blow to Poirier.

"It was a very discouraging time," he said. "But it was a learning experience."

Poirier and his team started over, redesigning the pump, replacing synthetic mechanical valves with pig heart valves, and improving connections where the pump joined the heart and its vessels. Nine years passed before they attempted another human trial, and this time it was a success. In clinical trials from 1985 to 1994, surgeons implanted the HeartMate in one hundred patients waiting for heart transplants. End-stage heart failure patients with an LVAD did much better after the transplant than patients who had not received the device. In 1994, a quarter century after Poirier began working on the LVAD, the FDA approved it as a bridge to heart transplant.

Poirier is chief scientific adviser to Thoratec, the firm that acquired Thermo Cardiosystems and now makes the HeartMate. Thoratec is working on a new generation of pumps that will be far smaller than the current HeartMate, will last for a decade or longer, and may be powered by electricity that is transferred through the patient's skin, eliminating the need for an opening in the patient's body. Poirier said that, should such devices come on the market, many of the 100,000 people who now die annually from end-stage heart failure could be saved.

"My hope is that these new devices become as common as pacemakers are today," said Poirier. "For that to happen they have to be smaller, more efficient, and less expensive. The whole industry is going that way."

Poirier's chief concern today is that a lengthy process of FDA approval makes it exceedingly difficult to bring new technologies to market. He noted that by the time the HeartMate was approved in 1994, many of the pump's components were already becoming obsolete. He contends that the FDA needs a method for expeditiously approving lifesaving technologies like the HeartMate, especially when the alternative is the death of critically ill patients.

"It's very discouraging," said Poirier. "A lot of technology never gets out there. It takes so long and costs so much that people will not do it. I am glad the FDA is there, but there has to be a middle ground."

Nevertheless, for Poirier the invention of the HeartMate has been the achievement of a lifetime and an example of what can happen when engineers work with doctors to tackle a critical health problem.

"I am an engineer and I like solving problems," said Poirier, who is 63. "And being able to help desperately ill people has been very satisfying."

Biomedical engineers at the University of Virginia are motivated by similar desires, but many are working not on devices but on the genetic and molecular processes that underlie heart disease. A principal area of focus is arterial disease.

Many people have a misconception about how plaque forms in the body's vessels, imagining that arteries are like pipes and that atherosclerosis is little more than fat clogging the pipes. Plaque does not, in fact, form that way but rather develops through a far more complex process. In effect, fatty cells in the bloodstream initially penetrate the inner layer of the artery's walls, known as the endothelium, creating small, fatty streaks. The single layer of endothelial cells sitting atop those streaks then emit chemical signals that attract white blood cells, whose job it is to seek and destroy bacteria, foreign organisms, or debris from dead cells. These white blood cells hear the call of the inflamed lining of the artery and, like cars approaching the scene of an accident, slow down before coming to rest above the fatty streaks.

The white blood cells then burrow through the endothelial layer and start to gobble the fatty streaks, or lipids. They gorge to the point where they can no longer digest all the fatty cells. Soon, the white cells—primarily monocytes and neutrophils—eat themselves to death and burst, creating a gooey mess known as foam cells. More white blood cells, zipping by in the bloodstream, are called to action, penetrate the artery's inner lining, eat more fat cells, die, and create an even greater mess just under the vessel's endothelial layer. (The *athero* in atherosclerosis is Greek for "paste." *Sclerosis* means hardness, which is what eventually happens to many plaques.)

"All these dead foam cells form the necrotic core of the plaque," said Brian P. Helmke, an assistant professor of biomedical engineering at U. Va. who is studying this process. "This accumulation of foam cells builds up and all the while you have the endothelial cells sitting on top of this mounting trash heap."

As the trash heap, or plaque, expands, it poses two grave risks to the body. One risk is that it can grow to the point where it completely blocks the artery, causing a heart attack or stroke. The other risk, which is an even likelier scenario, is that as the glob of plaque grows into the artery, the stretched and weakened inner layer of cells—the endothelium—gives way under the pressure. When it does, the rotten clump of plaque spills out into the artery, which instantly attracts clotting cells. The ensuing clotting around the disgorged plaque blocks arteries and causes heart attacks or strokes. This phenomenon also helps explain why half of all heart attacks occur after clots form in vessels that were less than 50 percent blocked.

A crucial link in this disease chain is when the endothelial cells lining arterial walls signal to the white blood cells to slow down and stop at the scene of this expanding plaque buildup. This so-called adhesion cascade is what sets the whole process of atherosclerosis in motion, and biomedical engineers realize that if they can block white blood cells from heading to the site of small fatty streaks, they might be able to keep plaques from forming. The adhesion cascade is a biological phenomenon. But analyzing the signaling that takes place among cells and the way in which white blood cells travel through arterial walls is a sophisticated exercise that engineers are undertaking with the help of robust computing and imaging power.

Klaus Ley, a physician who is also a professor of biomedical engineering and director of U. Va.'s Cardiovascular Research Center, is a world leader in investigating these initial phases of inflammation and plaque formation. The researchers in his lab are attempting to isolate and study the various parts of the adhesion cascade so they can figure out how to thwart it and fight not only heart disease but also such ailments as Crohn's disease, an inflammation of the lining of the colon.

A crucial element of Ley's research is the molecules involved in signaling white blood cells to peel off from the whirring traffic flow in the bloodstream and slow down at the site of plaque formation, a process known as "rolling." Using powerful microscopes trained on a patch of retractable, translucent skin near a mouse's scrotum, Ley's group has taken remarkable moving pictures of this process. You can see red blood cells and white blood cells speeding through the vessel in an indistinguishable blur. But along the vessel wall, white blood cells—also called leukocytes—have picked up a signal from the area of plaque formation and start to slow and then come to a stop. Eventually, they begin to squeeze through the vessel's inner layer to the nascent plaque below. The aim of Ley and numerous other researchers is to figure out which molecules are responsible for signaling the leukocytes to halt and then devise a way to block that signaling.

The ability to take and analyze videos of white blood cells inside a mouse's body has been a boon to understanding the genesis of plaque. And making sense of those videos would never have been possible were it not for exponential leaps in computing power, particularly in the past decade.

The person who has overseen this computer analysis at the University of Virginia is Scott T. Acton, an associate professor of electrical engineering. On a hot summer afternoon in 2004, I visited Acton in his lab at the engineering school, a complex of older brick buildings a short walk from U. Va.'s famed Lawn and Rotunda, designed by the university's founder, Thomas Jefferson. In an airy room, three of Acton's graduate students were working on the computer program that made it possible to identify and track individual white blood cells moving through a blood vessel.

Ten years ago, it took forty-five minutes to process just one frame of video taken of vessels in a mouse's translucent skin. By 2003, Acton's group could process a frame per minute. And by 2004, Acton could process 100,000 frames per hour. The machine that made this possible was a yard-high white box with the combined computing power of nine Intel Pentium 3 processors and eight Apple G-4 processors. Working with such technology, Acton's group has spent years perfecting a program that identifies the slowing white blood cells and outlines them on the computer screen. This enables Ley and his researchers to get detailed information about the speed and position of leukocytes—which have a diameter about a fifth that of a human hair—as they worm their way through the artery's inner layer of cells.

Such is the direction in which biomedical engineering is heading. The goal is to move beyond devices and engineer the biological foundations of life. Meanwhile, as the biological and genomic revolutions speed ahead, traditional technology—pacemakers, pumps, defibrillators—continues to save and extend the lives of millions of people.

Cardiac surgeon Curt Tribble is hopeful that more compact, longer-lasting left ventricular assist devices will be on the market within the next decade. "The pump's too big now," he said. "It doesn't need to be that big. It's gigantic. All it really needs to be is a cylinder about 1 inch by 3 inches. And we ought to have a device that lasts ten to fifteen years."

The longest a patient has survived on a HeartMate LVAD is a little more than three years. Still, a study of 129 patients at twenty transplant centers around the United States showed the undeniable benefits of these devices to people with end-stage heart failure. Fifty-two percent of patients with LVADs lived more than one year, while only 25 percent of patients being treated with conventional drug therapy lived a full year.

The world of cardiac devices and cardiovascular biomedical engineering is in a state of rapid flux these days. It is now clear that human transplantation will never come close to meeting the demand for new hearts, livers, and kidneys. As Tribble told me, "The honest truth is that transplantation is not our future."

It is also equally clear that entire mechanical hearts offer far less promise than originally believed. The long, difficult deaths suffered by Barney Clark and other recipients of the first mechanical hearts were attributed to the travails of pioneering devices. But two decades later, fully implantable mechanical hearts were still plagued by major problems: they tended to produce clots, experience mechanical failures, and destroy blood when it was forced through powerful machines. In early 2005, one of the most publicized mechanical hearts—the AbioCor, produced by Abiomed—was in deep trouble, with thirteen of fourteen patients who had received the heart dying during the course of medical trials. Scientists had been working on the AbioCor heart for twenty-two years.

Tribble believes the future of mechanical heart devices lies with the continuing refinement of LVADs. Like Poirier, he predicts there will be "massive growth" in the use of improved LVADs as a therapy for thousands of patients who don't receive human heart transplants. One ventricular assist device with great potential involves the use of magnetic suspension to hold a propeller-like "impeller" inside a cylindrical pump. The force of opposing magnets holds the impeller in place. Powered by electrical current that passes through a patient's skin, the impeller would pull blood out of the left ventricle and drive it up into the aorta. One of the developers of this axial flow pump is U. Va. mechanical engineer Paul Allaire, in conjunction with Utah inventor Don Olsen. Allaire's magnetically suspended pump, which has yet to be tried in humans, has several distinct advantages. It contains no bearings and thus could theoretically work inside a patient's body for many years. It is designed to produce few clots. And it is small, a little bigger than a man's thumb.

As cardiac devices improve, cardiologists like Jim Bergin are confident that cracking the genetic and cellular secrets of heart disease will simultaneously lead to new therapies. Bergin is particularly hopeful about the possibility of using stem cells to repopulate or replace damaged heart muscle.

"I'm 45 now, and I think that within my lifetime we'll see a number of these things come together," Bergin told me. "I hope that when I'm 65 or 70 and going on rounds with residents that when I say, 'There was a time when we transplanted entire hearts,' they'll say, 'What!' Because there may be so many new therapies. I think we'll be able to stop heart failure from being a major drain on the economy. It's now $24 billion a year. We should be able change one of the big causes killing people today."

Lurking behind all these undoubted advances in cardiac biomedical engineering is an important question: What will it cost? What if left ventricular assist devices one day become far smaller and more durable? Will tens of thousands of Americans who now die each year of heart failure get a new life? Left ventricular assist devices could one day become far smaller and more durable, and tens of thousands of Americans who now die each year of heart failure could get a new life. Such a development would be a major medical advance. But a health care expert cited by the *New York Times* said that should LVADs become as common as kidney dialysis—which keeps 300,000 Americans alive every year—the cost to insurers and Medicare could be $15 billion to $24 billion annually.

Roxanne Emswiler's HeartMate operation cost about $150,000, including the $65,000 price tag of the pump. But how to put a price on what the device accomplished? It not only saved her life but then sustained it for sixteen months as she awaited a new heart. For some patients, the LVAD is a "destination" therapy, meaning they are ineligible for a heart transplant and receive a ventricular assist device to give them a few more years of life. But Emswiler was a classic recipient of an LVAD as a "bridge to transplant," meaning it would tide her over until a donor's heart could be found.

Living with the pump, with its wires poking out of her body, was not easy. She and her husband, Larry, had to clean and dress the opening four to five times a day to prevent infection. At night, as the Emswilers slept, the pump rocked the bed. It took Roxanne hours, instead of minutes, to get ready to go out to dinner. When she did leave the house, she was tethered to the pump's external apparatus and a heavy holster of batteries. The LVAD produced a clot that caused her to have a small stroke, from which she has fully recovered. Still, she was grateful to the makers of the LVAD and the doctors who had placed it inside her.

"I look back at it now and I don't know how I did it," said Emswiler, who has two children. "My life depended on this machine. It was scary. But I was just so happy to be alive. This is the hand I was dealt and I made the best of it. I did what I had to do. I had to beat this thing."

On August 6, 2001, a donor heart at last became available, and Emswiler underwent an eight-hour operation. She stayed in the hospital eleven days and then was released to begin a new life.

Today, Roxanne Emswiler—a lively 52-year-old woman with short brown hair and wire-rimmed glasses—is in good health and has adjusted well to the immunosuppressant drugs she must take to keep her body from rejecting a donor heart. She is back at work at the bank with a profound respect for medical technology and a new outlook on life. The LVAD that kept her alive sits on a table in her living room.

"In my prayers I thank God for having people with that kind of knowledge to do that kind of work," Emswiler told me after one of her regular checkups at the University of Virginia Hospital. "I don't remember the last time I didn't go out and listen to all kinds of birds singing. I don't know if I'm going to be here tomorrow, and I tell people what I need to tell them. It's hard for me to keep my mouth shut when someone comes to the counter at the bank and starts griping about something minor."

Her husband added, "I certainly don't take her for granted. I used to just think we'd get old together. But not everybody gets old."

Chapter 5

To Breathe Again

The body can betray a person in myriad ways and at many speeds. Some illnesses—atherosclerosis, Parkinson's, Alzheimer's, numerous cancers—come on gradually, gathering force until a patient is firmly in their grip. But other afflictions hit with lightning speed, changing a person's life in an instant. Of these conditions none is more devastating, or more sudden, than a spinal cord injury. One moment a person is healthy, and the next—after diving into a shallow lake, surfing a big wave, or being thrown from a horse—he or she is on the ground, unable to move his or her arms and legs or perhaps even breathe. Spinal cord injuries are particularly cruel because they often happen to young people who, oblivious to the fragility of the human body and the tenuousness of life, push their luck to its limits and beyond. It is also cruel because the options for helping paraplegics and quadriplegics have traditionally been so limited. Indeed, regenerating the spinal cord is one of the most complex challenges facing medicine today.

One city, however, has become a Mecca for the treatment of spinal cord injury patients. People flock to Cleveland, Ohio, because biomedical engineers at Case Western Reserve University have spent decades working closely with physicians to give movement and bodily functions back to those who have been robbed of them.

During three weeks in Cleveland, I met many people who had sustained spinal cord injuries. Some had lost the use of their hands, others of their arms and hands, and still others of their entire body.

But the loss of movement in limbs is just one of the shattering consequences of a spinal cord injury. When a damaged spinal cord severs the connection between the brain and the body, a person often loses the ability to do many other things: to feel when it's time to urinate, to function sexually, and even to breathe. Such was the case with Laszlo Nagy, a 38-year-old stockbroker whose injury occurred so high on his spinal cord that—like the late Christopher Reeve—his brain could not send a message to his diaphragm to fill and empty his lungs with oxygen.

Until the night of June 24, 2002, Nagy was sailing through life, enjoying the pleasures of a middle-class American existence. After graduating from Cleveland State University, he moved to Chicago and began work as a stockbroker. He got married and in his spare time pursued his passion—riding Harley-Davidson motorcycles. Indeed, on the night of his accident, he had appeared on television to talk about motorcyclists' rights, which included, he argued, the right not to wear a helmet. He then met with a group of motorcycle buffs and, shortly after 11 p.m., agreed to give a woman a ride into downtown Chicago on a 2002 Harley Road King. Wanting Nagy to go faster, the passenger reached around to grab the throttle, which caused Nagy to lose control of the Harley. The motorcycle collided head-on with a Cadillac, sending Nagy into the car's windshield. In conventional parlance, we would say Nagy broke his neck, but that is not quite right. The force of the impact did not snap or sever his spinal cord but rather so badly wrenched it that the trauma and subsequent swelling and scarring meant that the cord could no longer serve as the body's conduit for nerve transmissions. Unconscious, unable to breathe on his own, Nagy arrived at the hospital without a heartbeat. In the emergency room, doctors yanked him back from the brink by shocking his heart to life and placing him on a respirator. (The passenger survived the accident with a broken pelvis.)

When he regained consciousness days later, Nagy said he "went nuts," unable to accept the incomprehensible: at age 36, he could move nothing below his neck. Months of rehabilitation and physical therapy followed, and Nagy—a youthful-looking man with dark hair, blue eyes, and a medium build—contemplated the question that every person with a severe spinal cord injury ponders: Was life really worth living in such a state?

But Nagy found the inner strength to keep going. Even after the breakup of his marriage—a common occurrence in the event of spinal cord injuries, as such a profound disability irretrievably changes relationships—he kept plowing ahead. Nagy learned how to maneuver his wheelchair by blowing into a strawlike device that translated his ventilator-powered breaths into motion. He transferred to a nursing home and then, after his divorce, moved in with his parents in Cleveland. He made plans to continue his work as a stockbroker.

Yet among the innumerable things he could no longer do, among the many shackles of his new life, one thing was particularly onerous: his ventilator, a machine that pumped air into his lungs through a tracheostomy in his throat.

"The ventilator was just utter hell," Nagy told me as we sat in a student lounge at Case. "I had to look over at that big noisy machine with all these tubes coming out of it and know that that was all that was keeping me alive. It had eighteen connections that could come undone at any time, and if there wasn't someone there who knew what they were doing, you were finished."

Being tethered to the ventilator also meant that when he left his house he had to worry about battery life. And because the ventilator bypassed his upper airway, which acts as a filter to the lungs, he was more prone to infections and respiratory illnesses. It also meant he couldn't smell a thing.

Deliverance from the ventilator came in June 2003 in the form of a technology that had been developed and perfected by biomedical engineers at Case. Building on centuries of experimentation with electricity and the body, Case engineers had for more than three decades been refining ways to use implanted electrodes to restore movement and function to paralyzed patients. Led by well-known biomedical engineer P. Hunter Peckham, a team of researchers had overcome numerous obstacles and discovered how to safely embed electrodes that enabled several hundred patients to lift their arms, grasp coffee cups and hair brushes, and even stand. It had been an arduous and unconventional journey, with the biomedical engineers even experimenting on themselves. Several still carry around vestiges of their early research into these so-called neuroprostheses: tiny electrodes embedded in the muscles of their arms, hands, and legs.

Several years before Nagy's accident, one of the original members of the group, J. Thomas Mortimer, had helped devise a new application for the Case technology, which is known as functional electrical stimulation (FES). Working first on laboratory animals and then moving into human trials, Mortimer and other researchers discovered that by implanting four electrodes in specific sections of the diaphragm, then hooking the electrodes up to an external power source, paralyzed patients could begin to breathe. By the end of 2004, nine patients had received these implants, known as diaphragm pacers. One was Christopher Reeve. And another was Nagy, who had the electrodes attached to his diaphragm on June 25, 2003, a year and a day after his accident.

Today, Nagy breathes on his own, ten breaths a minute, twenty-four hours a day, an advance that has freed him from the intrusive ventilator.

"That was the pivotal turning point of this whole thing for me," said Nagy. "I went off the ventilator and I took that first breath and it was incredible. You could smell again. I could smell perfume. It felt wonderful. I never looked back since, and I swear I'll never go back on the ventilator."

It also is saving insurance companies and taxpayers piles of money, as it cost $16,000 a month to keep Nagy on the ventilator. In addition, many people on ventilators need to be cared for in a nursing home, and only a limited number of such facilities can handle ventilator patients. An estimated 13,000 people in the United States and Europe are on ventilators and could benefit from the diaphragm pacer, according to Anthony R. Ignagni, a former Case engineer. He has joined Mortimer, who helped develop the diaphragm pacemaker, and two physicians to form a company called Synapse Biomedical Inc., which is now attempting to market the diaphragm pacemaker worldwide.

As Nagy and I spoke, Mortimer strode through the student center and walked over to say hello to Nagy. Mortimer praised Nagy for being one of the first patients to volunteer to try the diaphragm pacer. "It takes a lot of courage," said Mortimer.

"It was a pretty simple thing when you're faced with living on the ventilator," Nagy replied. "If I was still on it, I honestly don't know how I'd be today. I might still be in a nursing home. I probably would have caved in long ago."

Nagy's comment underlined another positive consequence of the diaphragm pacer, this one psychological. Perhaps the greatest battle that quadriplegics must wage is a mental one, and his liberation from the ventilator gave Nagy hope that this was only the first of a string of engineering and medical breakthroughs that might improve his condition. Like all people with severe spinal cord injuries, he dreams that tissue engineers and neurologists will one day discover a method of regenerating injured spinal cords.

"One of the biggest changes was the realization that they are doing things that help my condition," said Nagy. "Okay, now it's electronics, but then they will move into stem cells. The diaphragm pacer is a technological advancement that gives you hope there is more coming. One problem has been solved, and there are other solutions on the way."

Chapter 6

The Wires

A cure for Laszlo Nagy's underlying paralysis may still be a long way off. But using electricity to tackle a host of medical problems is gaining momentum. P. Hunter Peckham, J. Thomas Mortimer, and their colleagues are taking the techniques they developed for spinal cord injury patients and applying them to other conditions, such as incontinence, stroke-related paralysis, and obstructive sleep apnea.

One of the most intriguing frontiers of electrical stimulation, however, is in the body's most complex organ, the brain. A confluence of rapidly evolving developments—researchers' expanding knowledge of how the brain works, more precise imaging, and the development of ultrathin electrodes that can be implanted in the brain—has made brain stimulation, or pacing, a hot field. To date, the most progress has been made in treating movement disorders, such as Parkinson's and essential tremor. One of the nation's leading practitioners of brain pacing for Parkinson's is a surgeon at the Cleveland Clinic, Ali Rezai. Since 1997, he has implanted electrodes in the brains of more than 500 patients, most of whom had Parkinson's. The procedure, known as deep brain stimulation (DBS), is time consuming, requiring precise imaging and brain mapping. Picking a skilled surgeon is key. But DBS has proved to be highly effective, substantially reducing tremors in an overwhelming majority of people.

Rezai, who collaborates with biomedical engineers from the Cleveland Clinic and neighboring Case Western Reserve University, is confident that the use of deep brain stimulation for a wide variety of physical and psychiatric ailments is on the verge of rapid growth. The important thing is to identify centers of the brain that control different functions and then apply the proper charge—high frequency or low frequency, pulsating or steady—to counteract or block the malady. Researchers are now experimenting with ways to use DBS to prevent epileptic seizures, and Rezai thinks the technique could be used for pain control, autism, or improving function in people who have had strokes. On the psychiatric front, preliminary tests show that DBS may be helpful in treating obsessive-compulsive disorder. Rezai said that the technique may one day be used as a therapy for depression, addiction, and schizophrenia.

"Treating Parkinson's is just the tip of the iceberg," Rezai told me. "The future is very bright, and we can help many patients. This technique is evolving rapidly and will be coming on strong in the next decade. Think of it as being at a stage where heart pacemakers were in the 1960s."

Biomedical engineers are pushing the boundaries of brain research even further. Dawn Taylor, a biomedical engineer at Case and the Cleveland Veterans Administration Hospital, is one of a small group of investigators around the country making steady progress on a far-fetched dream: using an incapacitated person's thoughts to direct movement. By implanting an array of electrodes in a monkey's brain and then analyzing the firing of brain cells as the monkey moves, Taylor and others have succeeded in allowing a monkey to control a computer cursor simply by thinking about it. The goal is to enable people like Laszlo Nagy to move a robot arm, or an electrically stimulated muscle in a paralyzed arm, using only the firing of neurons in their brain. Some researchers are already beginning preliminary trials with people who have amyotrophic lateral sclerosis (ALS), also known as Lou Gehrig's disease, a degenerative nerve condition that eventually causes complete paralysis and death.

"We're looking at all kinds of options of how to move this into clinical reality," said Taylor. "Our goal in five years is to have it for ALS patients."

One of the biggest medical engineering successes in recent years has been the development of the cochlear implant, which uses an array of electrodes, speech processors, and transmitters to convey rudimentary sounds to the brains of deaf people. In the United States alone, more than 13,000 adults and 10,000 children have received cochlear implants. On a far more experimental level, researchers are trying to restore sight to the blind by using tiny cameras mounted on eyeglasses and semiconductor chips at the back of the person's eye to transmit visual signals to the brain. A device that actually restores some semblance of sight is years away, but the concept has promise and may one day come to pass.

All these electricity-based treatments—muscle stimulation, deep brain therapies, thought-controlled robotic limbs, semiconductors and electrodes to replace lost senses—have spurred talk in the press about the creation of a twenty-first-century "bionic man" pieced together at a high-tech lab bench. Some of this is plainly hype. Still, it seems certain that in the coming decades people with paralysis, deafness, or debilitating neurological disorders will benefit from harnessing a force—electricity—that has fascinated the medical field for centuries.

The first character, albeit fictional, to benefit from a bit of functional electrical stimulation was Mary Shelley's Frankenstein. Published in 1818, Shelley's novel *Frankenstein* drew on a growing body of scientific knowledge positing that electricity was the force that drove human thought and movement. The hunch that electricity might have therapeutic value goes back nearly 2000 years, to AD 50, when Scribonius Largus, physician to the Roman emperor Claudius, came up with a novel cure for leg pain: patients stood on wet sand atop an electric torpedo fish and received shocks from the raylike creature.

In the later half of the eighteenth century, after researchers learned how to store static electricity in a foil-filled capacitor known as a Leyden jar, physicians in Europe and America began experimenting on patients with electricity. As described by Ellen R. Kuhfeld, curator of scientific instruments at the Bakken Library and Museum in Minneapolis, a Swiss surgeon was able to restore function to the atrophied arm of a brain-damaged patient in 1748 by applying repeated electrical shocks that stimulated muscle movement. Around the same time, in Italy, medical professor Luigi Galvani and physicist Alessandro Volta performed experiments showing that electricity could stimulate the muscles of recently dead frogs. Galvani's nephew, Jean Aldini, obtained similar results while experimenting with executed murderers. Aldini also suffocated dogs and then revived their stilled heart by administering electric shocks. Even Ben Franklin made an unsuccessful attempt to treat paralysis with static electricity.

In the late nineteenth century and early twentieth, a host of electrical gadgets and devices came on the market to stimulate muscles or relieve pain. Most were instruments of quackery. But serious medical research into the uses of electrical stimulation continued, and by the mid-twentieth century biomedical engineers and physicians were making progress toward restoring some muscle movement in people with spinal cord injuries. In 1960, New York surgeon Adrian Kantrowitz affixed external electrodes to the buttocks of a paraplegic and, after applying a charge, was able to contract muscles that helped the patient briefly stand.

Then, in the mid-1960s, a handful of biomedical engineers intent on restoring some movement to paralyzed patients came together at Case Western Reserve University in Cleveland. Peckham arrived in 1966 as a young Ph.D. student. Trained in mechanical engineering at Clarkson University in upstate New York, Peckham had intended to study fluid flow and work in industry. But during his senior year he read an article in an engineering magazine about the design of heart valves. For Peckham, it was a turning point, as he realized that engineers could apply their skills to improve human health.

"At that point I sure as hell didn't know that you could make things and put them inside the body," recalled Peckham.

As he looked around the country at graduate schools, Peckham heard that engineers and doctors at Case were working together on numerous projects, including applying his field—fluid flow—to the cardiovascular system. Arriving at Case, he found that the extent of collaboration was even greater than he had imagined. Engineers and doctors had formed a group, known as Ampersand, to deepen their ties and find ways of bringing their two fields together to heal the sick. Peckham joined the group, making friends with the engineers and doctors who were taking the initial steps in functional electrical stimulation. Observing their work, he realized he had found his calling.

"I saw people who were into this idea of electrical stimulation, and it just captivated me," said Peckham. "And I found myself wondering, 'What am I doing studying fluid flow?' Once I saw how all these pieces could fit together, I knew there was a way to help people. I was really motivated by having the opportunity to see how this technology can be designed and developed and made applicable to give people independence. In my mind it was all about giving people back their freedom."

At that time, the pioneer of functional electrical stimulation at Case was a Slovenian researcher, Lojze Vodovnik, who worked closely with Case professor Jim Reswick and Mortimer, then a graduate student. To figure out how to bring paralyzed muscles back to life, Vodovnik and his young disciples not only experimented with animals but also embedded electrodes in their own muscles using hypodermic needles. The engineers attached wires to the electrodes, and by applying different charges to different muscles, Vodovnik, Peckham, and the others began to figure out how to crudely mimic the human body's complex movements. Visitors to Vodovnik's labs were confronted with the somewhat alarming spectacle of professors and long-haired graduate students zapping themselves with bursts of electricity that caused their hands to clench into death grips and their shoulders to hunch and spasm.

"Vodovnik put electrodes in his shoulders, his arms," recalled Mortimer, who went on to train two generations of students in neural prosthetic work. "He would do anything to his body. We all had electrodes in us. It was almost as if this guy [Vodovnik] had an infection and he gave it to all of us. We were ready to be infected. He's the guy who set us on the path we're on today."

In addition to his research, Peckham spent six years in the late

1960s and early 1970s working as the only engineer on the spinal cord injury unit in Cleveland's Highland View Hospital. His time there gave him an appreciation for the devastating impact of these injuries and the difference that even modest improvements in patients' abilities—such as the capacity to grasp an object—could make.

From the beginning, Peckham and his colleagues faced two basic challenges: how to make paralyzed muscles move, and how to give a quadriplegic the ability to control those movements. In a healthy person, the simple act of picking up a pencil is an intricate symphony of numerous muscle movements. Trying to mimic that process meant identifying the proper muscles that needed to be stimulated and in what order. Then Peckham and his colleagues had to coordinate those movements in a way that, by making one motion, a paralyzed patient could simultaneously activate a suite of muscles.

Case's researchers also had to overcome daunting physiological hurdles. Chief among these was that the inactive muscles of paralyzed people atrophied and underwent a change in metabolism.

"The problem was muscle fatigue," recalled Peckham, who initially worked as a graduate student in Mortimer's Applied Neural Control Laboratory. "The muscles did not have enough strength. We had to prevent that fatigue and coordinate a group of muscles to work together. We had to stimulate multiple muscles and learn how to coordinate those actions to get a functional movement. We also had to have reliable technology that wouldn't harm muscle. So we had to come up with something that was fine yet strong and would last, what, fifty years?"

Through repeated experiments on animals, themselves, and some patients, Mortimer, Peckham, and the Case team began to learn some fundamentals of functional electrical stimulation. They learned that a slower stimulation of muscles reduced fatigue, that by contracting muscles properly you could build strength and improve metabolism, and that electrodes with coiled wires were far sturdier, and less apt to break off in the body, than electrodes attached to straight wires. It quickly became clear that attaching electrodes to the skin was not effective, and so in 1974 the Case engineers began using percutaneous electrodes that penetrated through the skin to muscle. Peckham refined this system and, using six electrodes, was able to give some quadriplegics the ability to grasp objects with their hands, the patients controlling their movements either by making a slight movement with their wrists or by nudging an external joystick on their shoulders.

Eight years of study and experimentation went into the first system enabling patients to grasp. In effect, by giving back patients some use of their hands, the Case team was turning quadriplegics into paraplegics. But Peckham realized that he and his colleagues had to speed up the pace of their work.

"Here is something we had to learn," recalled Peckham, an avid sailor whose full head of brown hair, inexhaustible energy, and propensity to joke belie his age, which is 60. "When do you cut the apron strings? What's good enough? Rather than get things to perfection, at some point you had to get them to the patient. With these hand systems there are always things that need to be improved. But it's all about taking this research and translating it into clinical practice."

By the early1980s, another thing became obvious to Peckham and his colleagues. They had to move beyond a system that used electrodes attached to wires sticking out of a person's skin. Not only were the wires prone to break, but such a system was inconvenient for patients and required frequent cleaning and maintenance. So Peckham and his colleagues began working on a method of functional electrical stimulation using electrodes in muscle, with wires running inside the body to an implantable stimulator embedded in a patient's chest.

"We had to put it in the body and make it simple for the user," said Peckham. "That was the principle."

Their guinea pig was a young man named Jim Jatich, who in 1977 dove into a lake near Akron, Ohio, and damaged his spinal cord at the C-5 and C-6 vertebrae near the base of his neck, a common site for spinal cord injuries. The accident left Jatich a quadriplegic, although, like many quadriplegics, he could move his shoulders and had limited use of his upper arms. After spending a year at a rehabilitation hospital, during which time a fellow spinal cord patient committed suicide, Jatich resolved to overcome his injury. He met

Peckham, learned about his work with functional electrical stimulation, and volunteered to test the latest technology.

"I figured there was no sense crying or moping," said Jatich. "I wanted to see what was out there and do something about it. My attitude was, 'If I have a problem, let's figure out how we can make things work.'"

Jatich received his share of percutaneous electrodes, with doctors sticking them into his thumb, finger, or forearm to stimulate the contractions needed to grasp an object. Over time he received 150 percutaneous electrodes, and on one occasion he had 30 electrodes in his hand and arm.

"Oh, it was a bloody mess," said Jatich. "But I just kept coming back. I was interested, and I was willing to do anything. They would stimulate all the best muscles, and I would be able to pick up a pen and write and drink or brush my teeth in the lab. But when it was time to leave, they would pull the plug and I was paralyzed again."

Jatich became friends with Peckham and his colleagues, and when the time came to test an implantable system, Jatich was the natural choice. On August 26, 1986, orthopedic surgeon Michael W. Keith stitched eight electrodes to muscles in Jatich's forearm and hand and then tunneled the wires to his shoulder. There he implanted a matchbox-sized control device that enabled Jatich to raise his arm, reach, and grasp by moving his shoulder up and down.

Since then, Jatich has undergone several more operations, and he now has an updated twelve-electrode system in both arms that gives him even greater movement. Peckham and his fellow biomedical engineers have further refined the system's controls, so that Jatich and other patients can reach and grasp simply by making a slight wrist movement, which is then amplified by magnetic sensors. Known as the freehand system, it has provided Jatich with independence and freedom of motion, enabling him to live with his parents without burdening them, earn part-time income doing mechanical drawings on his computer, and even drive his own van with hand controls.

"How can you pay someone back for giving you the use of your hands?" said Jatich. "I've had the use of my hands for twenty years that otherwise I wouldn't have had."

Approved by the U.S. Food and Drug Administration in 1997 as a therapy for spinal cord injury patients, the freehand system has been implanted in 250 people, with many of the operations taking place at the Cleveland FES Center, where Peckham is director. (The FES Center is run jointly by Case, MetroHealth Medical Center, and the Cleveland VA Medical Center.) Peckham is disappointed that the freehand and other FES systems are not more widely used. A quarter million people in the United States have some form of spinal cord injury, with 10,000 new spinal cord traumas occurring in America every year. Half are paraplegics and half quadriplegics. Peckham said that many potential FES users are put off by having electrodes, wires, and control mechanisms embedded in their body. Others resist the surgery itself, which is costly—more than $50,000—and involves not only the insertion of the electrodes but also a separate procedure to transfer arm tendons, which improves motion. Most spinal cord injury patients still don't know that FES surgery even exists.

Perhaps the most important reason, according to Jatich and Peckham, is that many patients are waiting for researchers to find a cure—spinal cord regeneration.

"I talk to individuals who say, 'I'm going to wait. I'm going to wait,'" said Jatich. "But if it happens, I am exercised and ready for it. Plus, I wouldn't have my hand movement now, and I wouldn't know what to do without it."

These barriers have conspired to limit the use of FES systems and to doom a company, NeuroControl, that Peckham and Case colleagues formed to market the technology. But another company, NDI Medical—NDI is short for "new developments and innovations"—has emerged and is attempting to use FES systems to treat more widespread conditions, such as incontinence. NDI, along with the FES Center, was one of several entities to receive a $7.8 million grant from the state of Ohio to develop and market FES technology.

"Where we have succeeded is that we developed significant technology that is innovative and transferable to the clinic," said Peckham. "We've done it safely and no one has been hurt. We've based it on sound scientific principles. Where we've failed is we still haven't developed a sound commercial strategy. But we're working on that.

. . . We're looking at what has applicability not only to the disabled community but to the broader patient community."

The Cleveland FES Center continues to regularly implant neuroprostheses in paralyzed patients with a wide variety of injuries. The most common operation is implanting the freehand system, and on a chilly December morning in 2003, I witnessed orthopedic surgeon Mike Keith insert the latest twelve-electrode version in Annette Coker. A 45-year-old mother of two, Coker was returning from a Toledo Mud Hens baseball game on August 2, 2002, when she fell asleep at the wheel of her pickup truck 2 miles from home. Waking with a start as she drifted off the two-lane road, she whipped the wheel and lost control of the truck, which careened into a field. The pickup rolled over, and Coker, who wasn't wearing a seatbelt, was tossed violently around the cab. She broke her vertebrae at the C-5 to C-6 level and wrenched her spinal cord. Coker could still breathe but was paralyzed from the chest down.

"I knew exactly what I'd done, and when my friend [fellow passenger] came up to me, I said, 'Don't touch me! Let me die!'" recalled Coker, who had been working as a trainer of dogs to assist the handicapped. "There was a tingling, and I couldn't move, and I honestly thought for a minute or two that my body had been cut in half. I could shimmy my shoulders a little, and at that point I knew I was paralyzed."

Evacuated by helicopter to a Toledo hospital, she was placed in an MRI machine to evaluate the extent of her injury. A nurse held her hand, but she couldn't feel it.

"I kept thinking, 'This is a dream. I want to wake up. I want to get out of here,'" recalled Coker.

After nine days she was moved to a rehabilitation hospital. Her marriage of twenty-three years disintegrated. But she still had her two teenaged children, and she found the grit to keep going and the desire to once again lead an independent life. She had limited movement in her shoulders and upper arms and could barely move her hands. Coker knew that regaining function in her hands was critical to leading a semblance of a normal existence, and so when she heard about the Cleveland FES Center, she was eager to join Peckham's group of pioneering patients.

I first saw Coker in the operating room—or rather I saw Coker's arm, as the rest of her was shrouded under blue sterile paper. Dr. Mike Keith had opened a 4-inch incision in her left forearm, and he touched a long, narrow electrical probe to a glistening, crimson muscle. Keith then turned up a knob to administer a charge, and Coker's hand came to life, its fingers clutching together, then contracting and bending to touch her palm.

"That's a beautiful response," said Keith, who then measured the precise location of the probe so that an electrode could be sewn to the muscle at that spot. Fifteen people watched the operation, some assisting with the surgery and others—mainly biomedical engineers—helping Keith test the electrodes. The surgeon has worked closely with Peckham and his team for twenty years, and with Coker's operation they were working out the kinks in the new twelve-electrode version. Coker was the second patient to receive it.

Through a small incision in Coker's wrist, Keith placed the wand-like experimental electrode on another exposed band of muscle and turned up the electricity. This time, Coker's thumb contracted inward, as if to grasp something in her index finger. Keith then sewed an electrode to that muscle before turning his probe loose on yet another muscle, which, when stimulated, moved Coker's paralyzed index finger into position to meet her thumb—a move that would eventually allow her to hold a pencil.

On it went, for more than half a day, with Keith using electricity to bring Coker's muscles to life. When he was done with her forearm and wrist, he gathered together half a dozen wires and threaded them through a long, yellow plastic tube. Then, making the surgical transformation from grace to strength, he began shoving the tube up under the skin of her arm, toward her shoulder. Ultimately, the wires from all twelve electrodes would run through this conduit to her left chest, where a credit-card-sized device would translate Coker's various wrist motions into half a dozen movements that would give her the ability to raise her arm, sweep it to the side, and grasp objects, be they large like a coffee cup or fine like a knitting needle.

Keith—a powerfully built man who spends his vacations fly-fishing around the globe—said that from the moment he met Case's biomedical engineering team he was drawn to its goal of restoring independence to spinal cord injury patients.

"When you see these people who look like our wives and daughters and sons and in a tragic nanosecond their lives change . . . you want to do what you can to help," said Keith. "Spinal cord injury patients are devastated by the loss of independence and the helplessness that this injury inflicts upon them. We realized that if you were going to help people you had to give them greater independence. That's one way rehabilitation is measured—the lack of dependence on people. We realized that if we could give them help we could turn quadriplegics into paraplegics, and paraplegics are active and at large all around our country.

"When you give them back their hands they can do things like writing letters, making telephone calls, feeding themselves. They can get out and socialize more and be closer to normal. When you see a woman who had to be fed in a nursing home and after an [FES] operation she can go home and take care of her children and regain custody of her children, that's a good feeling."

Coker is not there yet, but in the summer of 2004, six months after her operation, she was planning to have the FES system implanted in her right arm and to eventually gain enough independence to leave the nursing home where she was living. Prior to her operation, she could make a feeble attempt at eating if a fork was strapped to her hand. But now, by making a slight motion with her wrist, her hand locked into place, allowing her to hold a fork on her own. When she finished eating, she made a slight upward movement with her wrist and her hand unlocked.

Sitting in her private room at a nursing home in Whitehouse, Ohio, Coker reached out, grabbed a bottle of spring water, and poured it into a glass—something she could never do before. She can also hold a pencil.

"I can write," said Coker, a slender, attractive woman with short brown hair. "I can brush my teeth. It's wonderful. Writing was out of the picture before. I can go to the store and pick things up off the shelf. I can adjust my clothes, apply lip balm. The other day I accomplished putting on my own sweatshirt. I can go to a restaurant and hold my own cup, which helps, because since the accident going to a restaurant has made me feel self-conscious. I think it's definitely brought me out of my self-consciousness a little. Just the fact that I can do stuff by myself makes me smile. I've definitely not reached independence, but I have a lot more than I had before."

When she leaves the nursing home, Coker will be aided by her specially trained dog, which can perform tasks such as helping her pull off her sweater, opening the refrigerator door, and removing clothes from the dryer and placing them in a laundry basket. She wants to drive and maybe even return to her prior job as a trainer for Assistance Dogs of America.

Visiting Coker at the nursing home, I realized how important the FES system was not only for her physical well-being but also for her mental health. In the space of two years, she had gone from being a vibrant, physically fit mother deeply involved in her children's lives to a divorced, wheelchair-bound resident of a nursing home. Despite her courage and inner strength, she was still overwhelmed at times by despair and distraught that she had been wrenched abruptly out of her children's lives. In 2004, her 20-year-old daughter, Terri, was studying to be a veterinary technician. Her son, Kyle, 18, was an engineering student at the University of Toledo.

Her eyes filling with tears, Coker told me, "When they're here, they're helpful. But they're at a busy age. If I was at home, I would at least see them. Our house was like Grand Central Station, and I miss all that hubbub. Not being at home and not seeing them often, it just drives me crazy. My daughter and her boyfriend bought a house. I would have liked to have been there to help, to hang curtains and scrub the floor."

However, the prospect of soon having the use of both hands is a lifeline for Coker.

"Human nature just tells you that you can't give up," she said as I prepared to say goodbye to her at the nursing home. "I can't handle being depressed, and I just tell myself that I will get out of this situation. Everyone kept telling me I was left on this wonderful earth for a reason. I want to get more independent, and if I can try out this new technology [FES] and help others in my predicament, I'm game."

The biomedical engineers and physicians at Cleveland's FES Center have gone well beyond restoring arm and hand movement to quadriplegics. One experimental system has enabled twelve paraplegics to rise from their wheelchairs, stand, and even walk a limited distance. Some Case biomedical engineers are working on systems that make swallowing easier for people who have had strokes; nearly a third of the 770,000 Americans who have strokes each year have trouble swallowing because of a loss of muscle control. Still other researchers at Case are studying ways to stimulate muscles and nerves in the throat to treat obstructive sleep apnea, a condition affecting tens of millions of Americans and one that can cause long-term health problems, including heart ailments.

Another use of electrical stimulation is to help spinal cord injury patients empty their bladder and, with less success, their bowels. Licensed under the trade name VOCARE, the technology has been implanted in about a hundred patients in the United States.

"This is a huge problem that is not talked about, and it is an area with huge societal and health impact on the patients," said Peckham. "It's a great indignity."

Graham Creasey, an English surgeon and bladder control researcher who has worked at the FES Center since 1990, takes his inspiration from a man who revolutionized the care of spinal cord injury patients worldwide. He was Sir Ludwig Guttman, a German Jewish émigré who moved to England before World War II. Until that time, virtually all quadriplegics and many paraplegics were hidden away and left to die. Many perished quickly from urinary tract infections, caused when urine repeatedly backs up from the bladder into the kidney. Others died of pneumonia and still more from rampaging infections stemming from the ulcerated pressure sores that developed on the back and buttocks of immobilized spinal cord injury patients.

But Guttman humanized the treatment of such patients, arguing that rather than being warehoused and left to perish, they should be given proper care, exercise, and hope for the future. Working at Stoke Mandeville Hospital in England, he began a program of rehabilitating soldiers whose spinal cords had been severed or injured during

World War II. In 1948, he initiated the Stoke Mandeville Games for paraplegic patients, which in 1997 became the World Wheelchair Games. Thanks to people such as Guttman, death rates among spinal cord patients are far lower today. Still, quadriplegics remain highly susceptible to fatal urinary tract infections and pressure sore infections, as evidenced by the death in October 2004 of Christopher Reeve from complications of an ulcerated bed sore.

CHAPTER 7

Moving into the Brain

Kathleen Schuessler came to Dr. Ali Rezai in the spring of 2004. A 66-year-old widow and former computer programmer from Mountain Home, Arkansas, she had been having tremors for thirteen years. They began with her right leg bobbing rapidly up and down. The tremors then spread to her right arm and eventually to her left leg. By 2004, even her left arm had started to shake. Like all people with Parkinson's, her symptoms arose after neurons in a portion of her brain, known as the substantia nigra, began to die off or malfunction in large numbers. The substantia nigra produces the brain chemical, or neurotransmitter, known as dopamine, which enables the body's muscles to function in a fluid, coordinated manner. About 1.5 million Americans have Parkinson's disease, with 60,000 new cases diagnosed annually. To varying degrees, these people experience tremors, rigidity, slowing motor ability, and balance problems.

Over the years, Schuessler had tried medicines, such as levodopa, that restore dopamine to the brain. But medications only slightly eased her symptoms, and by 2004 she was desperate for relief. She had difficulty eating or holding a cup because of her quavering hands. She couldn't enjoy two of her favorite hobbies, needlepoint and painting. Driving had become exhausting and difficult.

"My energy was at a very low level," Schuessler told me the evening before her surgery at the Cleveland Clinic. "My feet hurt from being in motion all the time. I had leg cramps. I used to get up early to do work because the twitches—I call them twitches—weren't so bad. But now, as soon as I start moving around, they start. I can't hold a phone in my right hand anymore. And just driving 5 miles to the store is annoying and even hazardous. I never know when my legs might start cramping.

"I've had it up to here. I said to my son that I was not going to live like this, that I was not going to take it anymore. I told him I didn't want to wind up in his cellar shaking apart. What else can I do? I can't stand being like this. I'm losing my independence."

To date, the most effective treatment for Parkinson's has proved to be deep brain stimulation, and the Cleveland Clinic's Center for Neurological Restoration, led by Rezai, is a leader in the United States for DBS treatment of movement disorders. All the technologies employed in a DBS operation—the electrodes used to administer the stimulation, the imaging employed to map the patient's brain, and the electrical apparatus that reads the firing of the brain's neurons—are the result of advancements in biomedical engineering.

As Schuessler and I talked, she sat on the edge of her bed in a robe, her right leg pumping up and down so badly that the bed shook. Her right arm quaked rhythmically in her lap. She was more than ready for her surgery.

When I arrived in the surgical suite around 10 a.m. the next day, Schuessler was on the operating table, her right arm and both legs shaking. She was sedated but conscious, as she would be through most of the operation. Her skull was fixed into place by an 18-inch, semicircular stereotaxic device that would guide the electrodes to the proper region of her brain. Before the surgery, physicians had taken detailed magnetic resonance and computerized tomography images, which would give Rezai a meticulous, three-dimensional picture of Schuessler's brain.

Rezai—a trim, dark-haired 39-year-old with the abundant self-confidence common to neurosurgeons—in 1997 became the first American surgeon to perform the DBS operation for movement disorders. After an anesthesiologist gave Schuessler a fast-acting and short-lived anesthetic, a surgical resident picked up a high-speed drill and cored out a dime-sized hole on the right side of Schuessler's shaved head. Using the calibrations on the stereotaxic halo, the resident and Rezai lined up a narrow cannula through which the surgical team would slide the titanium- and iridium-tipped electrode—four-hundredths of an inch thin—into Schuessler's brain. The man in charge of inserting the electrode was Dr. Benjamin L. Walter, a neurologist, who, by turning a wheel attached to a control box, moved the electrode a few thousandths of an inch with every revolution.

Except for a small spotlight on Schuessler's skull, the operating room was darkened, enabling Rezai and his team to see the computerized images. It was quiet, as well. And then, out of the silence, came the sound of Schuessler's brain. As the electrode moved into the nucleus of one of her brain cells, a static crackling filled the room and the lines spiked on an oscilloscope. Walter moved the electrode deeper, and it sidled up to another nucleus that spit out electrical signals and static, which represented Schuessler's thoughts and movements.

"The whole brain is one big ball of electricity," Rezai remarked.

He and Walter were initially targeting a jelly-bean-sized chunk of the brain known as the subthalamic nucleus. And within that area, they were searching for a far smaller area, only three-hundredths of an inch, that would enable them to still Schuessler's tremors. They knew precisely what they were looking for and would know it when they hit it. But in a testament to how little scientists still understand the brain, neither Rezai nor any neurosurgeon understands exactly why an electric charge in that region quiets Parkinsonian tremors.

Chance played a major role in the discovery that DBS therapy could alleviate the symptoms of Parkinson's and other movement disorders. In 1985, at the University of Grenoble, French neurosurgeon Alim-Louis Benabid was performing a last-resort procedure on a Parkinson's patient in which a part of the brain is destroyed by heat or electricity. Benabid was using an electrode to map the correct spot for destruction. As he pushed the electrode toward the thalamus and administered a shot of electricity, the patient's tremors abruptly ceased. Benabid had stumbled upon a major treatment for people with severe Parkinson's disease.

Benabid continued experimenting with the technique, performing the first official DBS procedure on a person with Parkinson's in 1987. Rezai later trained under Benabid at the University of Grenoble, where a long-term study of 148 patients has shown a marked improvement in their symptoms.

Cameron C. McIntyre is a biomedical engineer trained at Case Western Reserve University who is now at the Cleveland Clinic studying the effect of electrical stimulation on neurons. He said several hypotheses have been proposed to explain why DBS is effective in treating some movement disorders. Perhaps the most intriguing is that, in a diseased state brought on by a lack of dopamine, the affected neurons exhibit a rhythmic bursting activity. When a high-frequency electrical charge is applied to these pathological cells in the subthalamic nucleus, the current may, in effect, override the bursting and cause the cells to fire in a more normal way, thus reducing tremors.

In the operating room, where Schuessler's legs were trembling rhythmically on the table, Walter had advanced the electrode to the boundary of the subthalamic nucleus. He and Rezai knew they were approaching the sweet spot not only from the detailed imaging and computer mapping but also from extensive experience doing these procedures. A locus of much of the body's movement, the subthalamic nucleus is a hotbed of electrical activity, and the crackling sounds emanating from the speaker attached to the electrode began to intensify.

"We may be there," said Rezai. "We're knocking on the STN [subthalamic nucleus] door."

Moments later, they were in the subthalamic nucleus, and then in the region that controlled Schuessler's arm and leg movements. How did they know? Walter grabbed the patient's leg, and then her arm, and moved them vigorously, bending them at the elbow and knee. Every time he manipulated Schuessler's limbs, the firing of neurons in her brain exploded, sending out bursts of a static "zizzzz" and causing the electrical waves on the oscilloscope to spike.

"That's your brain talking," Rezai said to Schuessler.

"You hear that?" added Walter. "Every time I move your leg down, you can hear the neurons firing."

Walter moved the electrode deeper into her subthalamic nucleus, and suddenly the operating room was filled with a rhythmic, oscillating static, like the sound of a stuck record.

"You hear that?" asked Rezai. "That's a tremor cell."

Rezai and Walter had found the hot spot in Schuessler's diseased brain. It was quite a feat, one that Rezai had explained earlier in these terms:

"It's like you start in China and move west, travel through India, then go to Europe. You want to find Spain, so you go there, then you go to Madrid, and then you want a particular zip code in Madrid. You go there, then you go to a certain neighborhood, then a particular street, then an individual house. And then you go into an individual room in that house. That's what we do."

Rezai was exactly where he wanted to be, a place where every manipulation of Schuessler's ankle, knee, wrist, or elbow set off a spike of electrical activity. He explained to her that he was going to remove the recording electrode and replace it with a stimulating electrode. He would then begin sending an electrical charge to each of the four different contacts at the electrode's tip, seeing which contact, or combination of contacts, was most effective.

"Will my leg stop jumping?" asked Schuessler.

"That's the plan," replied Rezai.

Around 1 p.m., a technician wheeled an X-ray fluoroscope into the operating room. The machine would be used to track the progression of the stimulating electrode into Schuessler's brain. A surgical resident inserted the electrode, and Rezai watched as it slid into the center of a bull's-eye that had been marked on the fluoroscope. Meanwhile, Schuessler, who had been flat on her back for four hours, was drowsy, causing her tremors to subside somewhat.

"Okay, bring your tremor up for us," Rezai said to Schuessler, only half joking.

His words roused her, and then he asked her to count backward from one hundred in increments of three—an exercise designed to cause some tension and increase her tremors but also to make sure the stimulation was not affecting her speech. Soon, Schuessler's legs began quaking. Rezai gave the order, and Walter flipped a switch that sent a high-frequency charge into the patient's brain. As if on command, the tremor in her left leg—controlled by the right hemisphere in her brain—stopped shaking.

Rezai and Walter experimented with different voltages and combinations of contacts, settling on a two-volt charge as the most effective. Other than some tingling in her hand at a higher voltage, Schuessler said she felt fine.

"Very good, very good results," Rezai told her. "Now we're going to put you to sleep for a little while."

"Good," replied Schuessler.

With the patient unconscious, Rezai and his team drilled a small hole in her skull to begin treating the left side of her brain, which would quiet the tremors on her right side. Around 5:30 p.m., the DBS procedure was completed, more than eight hours after it began. A week later, surgeons implanted two small pacemakers below her collarbones. Wires ran from the pacemakers, under the skin of her neck and scalp, and into her brain. The strength of the charge could be adjusted by an external controller held next to the pacemakers.

Four months after her surgery, I spoke to Schuessler. Her tremors had almost entirely subsided, and she was able to sit still and read without shaking, draw and paint without her trembling arms and legs interfering with her art, and eat at restaurants without food falling off her utensils. She could drive with greater ease, although her right foot would begin to tremble if she was at the wheel too long.

"I'm much better," she told me over the phone from her Arkansas home. "I would say I'm 90 percent better. You don't know how much it means to be able to sit still and not shake. My neighbor can't get over how quiet my legs have gotten. They used to be popping out all over the place."

Long-term studies of DBS patients show similar results. A French study, which appeared in the *New England Journal of Medicine* in

2003, followed forty-nine people with Parkinson's for five years. Among them, motor function improved 54 percent after DBS surgery, the need to take tremor medicine declined, and most were able to live without a caregiver after the operation.

But the success of the procedure still depends heavily on the experience and skill of the surgeon, and Rezai said he periodically performs DBS procedures on patients whose electrodes have been improperly implanted at other hospitals. Rezai also said there is ample room for improvement in current technology, and he is hopeful that new inventions—such as miniature MRI transmitters that can be inserted in the brain—will improve accuracy and cut the time of the procedure by many hours. Companies like Medtronic, a leader in heart pacing, are now investing more money in developing better electrodes, pacemakers, imaging technology, and computer software for the brain.

"The technology we use now still has a long way to go," said Rezai. "It's archaic. It's very primitive, and things will be very different ten years from now."

As engineering and technological advances occur, and as neuroscientists learn more about diseases of the brain, Rezai and others believe deep brain stimulation may be used for a host of ailments, from obsessive-compulsive disorder to autism.

"It's a very exciting field to be in right now because we can affect many conditions that we have been unable to treat before," said Rezai. "This technology is evolving rapidly. I envision a day where we implant microchips and monitor various brain functions and then intervene to affect them. I see a future with a combination of multiple devices that sense a brain malfunction, then release electricity or a drug. These devices will detect a storm in the brain, like epilepsy, and intervene with a burst of electricity before it becomes a massive storm. We need a strong cross-fertilization with biomedical engineering. Biomedical engineering is absolutely critical to the future of neurosurgery in developing chemical, electrical, and sensing devices for the brain."

Rezai collaborates with scientists from Medtronic, which has sold more than 20,000 of the DBS systems for people with Parkinson's.

Medtronic researchers also are intrigued by the possibilities of using DBS to treat mental disorders and addiction. Knowledge of the brain is growing rapidly, and already neuroscientists have a good idea of which regions of the brain are involved in depression, anxiety disorders, compulsive behavior, and addiction. Rapid improvements in imaging also are allowing neuroscientists to see how the brain functions in real time, further enhancing science's ability to pinpoint the locus of psychiatric ailments. All these developments improve the chances of using DBS to treat psychiatric problems.

"Everything we think, do, and say is controlled up here," said Mark Rise, senior principal scientist with Medtronic Neurostimulation, pointing to his head. "So we try to manipulate the brain to treat these pathologies."

In a first step, Medtronic is supporting physician trials of roughly three dozen patients with obsessive-compulsive disorder (OCD). The patient sample is small, but Rise said that half the group reported significant benefits from deep brain stimulation.

The challenges of using deep brain stimulation are significant. One issue, said Rise, is targeting the area of the brain involved in a pathology without causing problems in adjacent regions. But electrical brain stimulation offers a decided advantage: it can be turned on and off, can be adjusted to match the volume of brain tissue being targeted, and appears to do no irreparable harm to the brain.

"It's a brave new frontier," said Rise. "Much of what we have discovered about the brain is because somebody tried something. And the more we learn about which neural circuits are associated with which aberrant behaviors, we'll be able to apply and modify different tools. And that's where biomedical engineering comes in."

At Case's Neural Engineering Center, director Dominique Durand is heavily involved in researching epilepsy and whether DBS may alleviate its devastating symptoms. Roughly 2.5 million Americans have epilepsy, which occurs when a synchronous firing of cells in a large portion of the brain overloads the organ's complex circuitry, causing seizures. (Coordinated firing of cells is essential in an organ like the heart but anathema to the brain, the site of an intricate, boisterous, and multilayered dialogue among billions of brain cells.) Roughly 15 percent of epileptics do not respond to conventional drug therapy, exposing them to unpredictable and potentially life-threatening seizures.

To date, deep brain stimulation has had mixed results combating epilepsy in animals and humans. In some experiments, inserting electrodes into a part of the brain—the anterior nucleus of the thalamus, where many seizures begin—and applying a rapid-fire, high-frequency signal has disrupted epileptic seizures. But because epilepsy occurs in various parts of the brain—a grand mal seizure erupts when synchronous neuron firing spreads to both hemispheres—it is tough to treat. In Durand's lab, graduate students are doing basic research on rat brains, applying electrical stimuli and drugs to neurons from the hippocampus, where epileptic seizures are often centered.

Medtronic is currently running a trial of 125 epilepsy patients to see if DBS can reduce the seizures. Although acknowledging the daunting challenges, Rise said electrical stimulation may one day prove to be an effective treatment for some epileptics. "If you know which cells are prone to start a seizure and have a system to detect seizures when they start, you could theoretically apply a stimulus and interrupt the seizures as they begin," said Rise.

The far frontier of biomedical engineering and brain research is now being explored at Case, the University of Pittsburgh, Duke University, and several other research centers. It involves a dream that once seemed pure science fiction but now is being realized in experiments with monkeys: enabling a paralyzed person to move a robotic arm, or his or her own electrically stimulated arm, simply by thinking about it.

Some of the leading research in this field is being conducted by Andrew Schwartz, a professor of neurobiology at the University of Pittsburgh. I visited Schwartz's lab and was fortunate enough to meet Pearce, a rhesus macaques monkey that stands about 2 feet tall, weighs 16 pounds, and has large brown eyes and pink ears. He also has a winning disposition and a penchant for hard work, which is why, on a September morning in 2004, postdoctoral fellow Beata

Jarosiewicz was wheeling him out of the primate dorm and into the laboratory, where he would happily toil for three hours in the interest of science—and a drink of water.

Dressed in a blue lab coat, Jarosiewicz pulled Pearce's cage into a small room equipped with a high chair, a computer monitor, wires and electronic boxes, and a small bottle of water with a metal spout. Pearce clambered eagerly into the chair, all the while looking fondly at Jarosiewicz and occasionally cooing to her, which prompted Jarosiewicz to reply, "Hey Pearcey!" Jarosiewicz immobilized the monkey's right hand by placing it inside a plastic tube and then attached an infrared sensor to Pearce's left hand. Next, she affixed a plastic cap to his head. The cap plugged into a device that was connected to sixty-four electrodes in Pearce's brain, each one-third the thickness of a human hair. Wires from the cap ran outside the room to a bank of computers and monitors where Jarosiewicz would soon sit.

Jarosiewicz closed the door. Inside the small room, lit only by a night light, Pearce waited for the action to begin. We watched Pearce on a television monitor, and he sat patiently in his chair, craning his neck and looking first toward the door, then toward a mirror that reflected a computer screen.

"Okay, Pearcey, give it a try," Jarosiewicz instructed.

The monkey began waving his left hand in the air. The movement of the infrared sensor on his hand was picked up by a camera, which then translated the motion onto the computer screen in front of Pearce. When the monkey moved his hand upward, a gold ball on the screen moved up, and when he nudged his hand to the left, the ball moved left. Pearce's task was simple. He had to superimpose the gold ball over a moving green ball on the screen, and he began to do so with ease. Every time he would successfully cover the green ball, a click would sound and a drop of water would automatically be released from the bottle into Pearce's mouth.

As Pearce performed his job a few dozen times, the electrodes protruding one-eighth of an inch into his brain also were doing theirs. The electrodes had been inserted next to neurons in Pearce's motor cortex, which gives the orders for muscles to move. Each of the many millions of neurons in the motor cortex has what scientists call a "preferred direction." That means that when a monkey or a person wants to move his or her arm to the left, all the neurons that prefer moving to the left will speak up and fire a signal, ordering the arm to go left. So when Pearce's brain decided he needed to move left to cover the green ball, the sixty-four electrodes, placed next to a sampling of motor cortex neurons, would take an electronic snapshot of the brain as it ordered that movement and would transmit that information to powerful computers at Jarosiewicz's work station.

Then the fun began. After obtaining a good electronic portrait of Pearce's brain ordering his arm to move in all directions, Jarosiewicz walked back into the room. Pearce's head whipped around to see what his handler was doing. Jarosiewicz then immobilized Pearce's left arm in a plastic tube and walked out.

Pearce once again sat patiently in front of the computer screen. The gold and green balls appeared. And then something remarkable happened. Pearce stared intently at the screen and, after a few tries, began superimposing the gold ball over the green ball simply by thinking about it. Indeed, for the next fifteen minutes, Pearce succeeded in placing the gold orb over the green orb 60 percent of the time—all by thinking the gold ball into the proper position.

What had happened? It was all the work of the electrodes, an intricate computer algorithm, and the neurons in Pearce's motor cortex. The computer already knew which way the majority of the monkey's neurons fired when he moved his hand left or right, or up and down. Pearce's hands may have been immobilized, but when he saw the two balls on the screen, his brain fired like crazy, trying to move the gold ball in a certain direction. The computer picked up that information from the electrodes, digested it, and translated it into a command for the gold ball to move in the direction Pearce was thinking. When his hands were, in effect, tied down, Pearce's neurons fired in a slightly different manner, but the computer program was still able to translate that electrical activity into a command to move in a specific direction. In this manner, Pearce was able to think a thought and have that thought translated into a computer movement.

Dawn Taylor, a Case biomedical engineer who did her Ph.D. work at Arizona State University under the supervision of Schwartz, told me earlier, "What's truly amazing is that there's this much learning and plasticity with animals doing this a few hours a week. Imagine if humans do this all the time, and how human cells will adapt and customize. The brain is so flexible and adaptive."

The goal is plain: to eventually implant such electrodes in the brains of spinal cord injury patients, or people with ALS, and enable them to command prosthetic devices or muscles controlled by FES electrodes. Indeed, in Schwartz's lab, researchers have devised a robot arm that would be attached to a computer, which in turn is connected to a monkey's brain. Already, Schwartz's group has had limited success in enabling a monkey to use a robotic arm to bring an orange into its mouth—all with thought control.

Other researchers around the country are now pursuing experiments like Schwartz's, with exciting results. They include John Donaghue at Brown University, Miguel Nicolelis at Duke University, and Philip Kennedy of Neural Signals Inc., of Atlanta, who has implanted electrodes in several disabled people that enabled them to type, using thought control, at a very slow rate. Kennedy and Schwartz are now collaborating and may be among the first to experiment with thought-controlled prosthetic systems in ALS patients, many of whom eventually become so paralyzed that they can do little more than blink.

But Taylor and others advise against euphoria or overly optimistic prognostications. For Schwartz, getting to the point where Pearce could control objects on a computer screen with his thoughts has been two decades in the making. It took him two years to come up with a technique that would enable the electrodes to remain stable in the monkey's brain. Schwartz and others are still grappling with the persistent problem of electrodes picking up firing from other neurons not involved in movement. Devising the computer algorithms that allow a monkey's thoughts to be translated into actions also has been devilishly complex. And electrodes need to be made thinner and more durable.

Still, among people like Schwartz and Taylor, there is a palpable sense that they are on the threshold of discoveries that one day will enable paralyzed people to do things about which they can now only dream.

"We have to get this into a stable, long-term implant," said Taylor. "Where it stops, who knows? To move this into humans has always been my goal. Enabling paralyzed people to think about something and do it is the Holy Grail."

Chapter 8

The da Vinci

To watch Dr. David D. Yuh of the Johns Hopkins Hospital perform an operation while sitting 15 feet from the patient is impressive indeed. But if Yuh's collaborators in the engineering school at the Johns Hopkins University have their way, the doctor's robotic surgery wizardry will soon look antiquated.

On a raw, windy winter morning in 2005, Yuh took up his station in an operating room adjacent to the hospital's Halsted building, an edifice named for the physician credited with helping to bring American surgery into the modern era. In the late nineteenth and early twentieth centuries, Dr. William Stewart Halsted, a professor of surgery at Johns Hopkins, introduced a host of changes—including the use of rubber gloves, sterile operating room techniques, new methods of anesthesia, and the creation of a comprehensive training, or residency, program for young surgeons—that helped transform a trip to the operating table from a frequently fatal experience into a sanitary, medical exercise that offered a good chance of survival. Halsted and the succeeding chiefs of surgery at Johns Hopkins, including renowned cardiac surgeon Alfred Blalock, also championed one of the axioms by which Yuh and generations of surgeons were trained: to attain, in Yuh's words, "maximum exposure," meaning to make an incision large enough so that there was ample room to get the hands inside the body, push aside the non-target organs, and get down to business on the diseased tissue.

This morning, Yuh was violating that principle as he took minimally invasive surgery, which older surgeons once disparaged as "minimally successful surgery," to new heights.

Yuh—who as a teenager invented a wildly successful video game (he prefers not to name the game, as he shudders to think of the countless hours adolescents have wasted playing it)—was seated in front of a console in the corner of the operating room. It was a large, gray machine that, truth be told, was roughly the size and shape of a video arcade game. His eyes were pressed against two eyepieces, his fingers and thumbs were attached with Velcro straps to handlelike controls that he maneuvered fluidly in space, and his feet pumped a couple of pedals up and down.

On the receiving end of this high-tech machinery was an 86-year-old patient with a heart problem. He was James Clark Jr., former president of the Maryland State Senate and a man slipping into heart failure because his heart had begun conducting electricity poorly. Unable to pump blood efficiently, his heart had tried to compensate by expanding from the size of a fist to the size of a grapefruit, the organ's walls gradually thinning as they ballooned. By the time Clark came to see Yuh, his heart was pumping only about 20 percent of the blood out of its left ventricle with each beat, as opposed to about 50 to 60 percent for a healthy person. As a result, the former senator felt fatigued, and fluid was accumulating in his legs.

"I wasn't a basket case by any means, but it was dragging me down," said Clark, a farmer from Howard County who served in the Maryland State Senate for twenty-four years and was its president from 1979 to 1983. "When your legs start swelling up like that, you know you're not doing too well."

No surgery could cure Clark's condition, but the implantation of a biomedical engineering device could help. It was a so-called dual-lead pacemaker, which—as opposed to traditional, single-lead pacemakers—would send a coordinated electrical pulse through both chambers of Clark's heart, helping it to pump with greater efficiency. Such pacemakers are usually implanted by threading the leads through a vein in the groin and into the heart. But Clark's anatomy, like roughly 20 percent of pacemaker patients, was quirky, and after seven hours of trying, cardiologists had implanted one lead but had given up trying to place the other lead in his left cardiac chamber. Then they turned to Yuh, who, at age 40, is one of Johns Hopkins's youngest cardiac surgeons and, as director of the surgical research program, the point man on collaborations with the Engineering Department.

Before the arrival of the da Vinci surgical robotic system at Johns Hopkins a few years before, Yuh would have performed a thoracotomy on Clark, which involves making a 4- to 6-inch incision along the left side of the chest, cutting through muscle, spreading open a couple of ribs, and attaching leads to the external surface of the heart. The operation would have inflicted a considerable amount of pain on Clark and required a significant recovery time.

Instead, Yuh turned to the da Vinci, the most widely used robotic surgical system in the world, with more than 210 installed in operating suites in the United States, Europe, and Asia. The precursor of the da Vinci was originally developed at the Stanford Research Institute, with funding from the U.S. Defense Department's Advanced Research Projects Agency (DARPA), which wanted to develop methods of performing remote battlefield surgery. In 1995, the three inventors—physicians Frederic Moll and John Freund and engineer Robert Younge—formed Intuitive Surgical, a California-based company that would eventually produce the da Vinci. Refined over the past decade with numerous patented technologies, the da Vinci consists of the surgeon's console and the robot, complete with three arms, that hovers over the patient. The da Vinci is increasingly being used in the United States for dual-lead pacemaker and heart valve operations, as well as for operations to remove the prostate, repair the esophagus, or perform gastric bypass for the obese. European surgeons have even used the da Vinci to perform coronary artery bypass operations, a robotic procedure now being done in the United States on a trial basis.

Yuh made four pencil-sized holes in Clark's left chest wall and inserted three robotic arms into the openings. The fourth hole would be used by Yuh's assistant, Gary Santmyer, to insert surgical tools into Clark's chest. Sitting at his console, Yuh—a man of medium height, slight build, and a warm, unassuming manner—manipulated controls that sent commands to the robot suspended above the operating table. The device then moved the robotic arms, with built-in lights, that were whirring around inside Clark's chest cavity, which had been pumped full of carbon dioxide to fill the space with gas to make it easier to maneuver the arms.

As Yuh explained, the da Vinci offers significant advantages over minimally invasive laparoscopic surgery, which also allows a surgeon to operate through small incisions using wandlike instruments. For one, the robot's hands do not tremble, making it well suited for fine suturing. And the da Vinci has a feature, known as EndoWrist, that smoothly translates the surgeon's gestures into robotic action. The da Vinci could perform numerous gestures better than laparoscopic tools, including a twisting motion vital to screw the corkscrew-shaped pacemaker leads into Clark's heart. The da Vinci's arms could be changed depending on whether Yuh wanted to grasp, cut, or suture.

Talking frequently with Santmyer, Yuh maneuvered the robot's cauterizing tool to cut through the pericardial sack surrounding the heart. Normally, Yuh—who uses the da Vinci system to perform several pacemaker implantations a month and also to repair defective heart valves—takes ten to fifteen minutes to screw in each lead. But Clark's lungs were abnormally voluminous and kept spilling over onto his cardiac tissue, making it difficult to operate. Yuh used the robot to hold back the lungs with a suture in the pericardial sac, but because the da Vinci gives surgeons no sense of how much force they are applying—a problem that biomedical engineers at Johns Hopkins and elsewhere are working to solve—Yuh broke the suture. Eventually, however, with Santmyer's help in controlling the sprawling lung tissue, Yuh managed to twist the half-inch corkscrew lead—attached to a quarter-sized piece of white mesh—into the heart muscle. The process took an hour, leaving Yuh briefly pining, perhaps, for the old days of big incisions and maximum exposure.

The second lead, a backup placed on a more accessible part of the heart, went in with ease. But as I watched the procedure on a TV monitor above the foot of Clark's bed, I spied another challenge that engineers at Johns Hopkins are attempting to surmount. Every time the former senator's heart beat, it would juke about an inch from side to side. Yuh wanted to place the lead near a large blue vessel on the surface of the heart, and a misstep, caused by the jumping heart, could have led to a dangerous nick in the vessel. Yuh screwed in the lead without complications, but Johns Hopkins engineers are working on robotic systems that will take the beating heart's motion into account and automatically place a lead, or make an incision, in a precise location on moving cardiac muscle.

After Yuh wrapped up the surgery in about two hours, he chatted in the corner of the operating room with two engineers from Intuitive Surgical. They asked him how he would improve their device, and he replied that he'd like a tool that would make it even easier to screw in the pacemaker leads. He also would like a fourth robot arm, which Intuitive had recently introduced. But Yuh was essentially pleased with the operation and the device and is excited to be a part of the effort to bring the tools of engineering and robotics even deeper into the world of surgery.

"I find it fascinating," said Yuh. "It's a new surgery and a new paradigm. Robotic surgery is still a modality looking for an application. Some things it does well, and some things not so well. But the da Vinci is just one step in a process of evolution, and it will probably not be here in its current form in five years. Surgical robots will become more specialty-driven, and you'll probably have one for the heart, one for GI [gastrointestinal]. And there won't be as much of a barrier to robotic surgery with a new generation of surgeons. We see younger surgeons who sit down at the da Vinci and are immediately comfortable with it."

A month after the operation, Clark was feeling better. His breathing came more easily, and he had far less fluid accumulating around his ankles.

"I think the results were good," he said in a phone conversation from his farm. "I have more energy. And I do right much walking now. I wanted them to get that thing [the dual-lead pacemaker] hooked up, and I didn't care how they did it. I still don't know how that robot was able to screw that thing in there."

Over the past half century, surgeons like Yuh have worked closely with engineers to vastly improve the quality and safety of surgery. This collaboration has led to such advances as the implantation of pacemakers and defibrillators, the development of artificial heart valves, the invention of heart-lung bypass machines for open-heart surgery, the advent of laparoscopic surgery, and the refinement of devices to safely deliver anesthesia. Similar progress has been made in the field of orthopedics, where the union of surgeons and engineers has made joint replacement surgery one of the most successful and common operations in the United States, with 175,000 hip replacement and 365,000 knee replacement surgeries performed annually.

At Johns Hopkins, a leader in biomedical engineering and surgical robotics, researchers are collaborating closely with surgeons on many fronts to bring surgery into the twenty-first century. Biomedical engineer Kam Leong, partnering with physicians in the Department of Neurosurgery, has helped devise a biodegradable polymer that is implanted in people with brain tumors and releases targeted chemotherapy agents over time. Allison M. Okamura, assistant professor of mechanical engineering, is working with Yuh to invent systems that will give surgeons an accurate idea of how much pressure they are applying when using robotic surgical systems.

Johns Hopkins also has created the Center for Computer Integrated Surgical Systems and Technology (CISST), which uses advanced imaging, computer modeling, and robotic technology to help surgeons more accurately plan and perform operations. Headed by Professor Russell H. Taylor, the center is devising systems, some of which are already in limited clinical use, that enable doctors to place radioactive seeds in prostate tumors with an unprecedented degree of accuracy, precisely zap liver tumors with radio waves during minimally invasive surgery, or use small robotic systems to operate on patients' throats or nasal passages.

"What we'd really like to do with these procedures is integrate imaging directly with surgical intervention," said Taylor. "What you're after is a partnership between surgeons and machines that will help surgeons do something better than they could otherwise do by themselves."

Taylor worked with Peter Kazanzides—the chief systems and robotics engineer at the CISST—to invent a system known as

ROBODOC, which uses robotic tools to precisely drill a patient's bones to ensure a tight fit for the prosthetic devices used in joint replacement surgeries. The system, in clinical trials in the United States, has been used in 15,000 operations in Europe, Korea, and Japan and employs a high-speed rotary cutter to drill bone right in the operating room.

The aim of Gregory D. Hager, a professor of computer science who collaborates with Taylor, is to give robots more intelligence and autonomy, rather than having them merely be an extension of a surgeon's hands, as they are now with the da Vinci system. Hager's vision is to develop coordinated imaging and robotic systems that will lead the surgeon to a precise spot inside the body and then, at the surgeon's command, execute a perfect incision or sew up a wound. (The robot could learn the ideal suturing technique by having a computer trace the stitching motions of a master surgeon and then transferring those gestures to the robot.) Image-guided robotic surgery, Hager believes, could also perform delicate operations on tiny vessels in the eye or brain, procedures now beyond the realm of human precision.

"I am trying to understand how to develop true surgical assistance," said Hager. "A lot of what we're talking about is what you could call 'skill amplifiers.' The da Vinci system does not understand anything about surgery. It takes signals from the surgeon and performs those inside the body. But what sort of intelligence can you put into that system to help the surgeon? Can you help the surgeon understand heart motion? Ultimately what will go on in surgery is that through imaging and computers there will be a playbook in which the robot will help the surgeon come in, locate the gall bladder, for example, and detach it. We will develop systems to observe the surgeon and assist the surgeon. For a lot of operations it may not make sense to have your hands in the patient. Automation may do it better than hands. I think the opportunities are enormous, and it's a question of making imagination meet reality."

Chapter 9

The Virtual Surgeon

Those inclined to employ a liberal definition of biomedical engineering might argue that its application in the realm of surgery and orthopedics began several thousand years ago when the ancient Egyptians invented a wooden finger prosthesis. The pirate's peg leg and hook hand were another crude step in the direction of prosthetics and artificial limbs. Until the twentieth century, surgery was about as rudimentary, and a trip to the operating table just as often killed patients, from surgical errors or infection, as cured them. One premodern doctor with the biomedical engineer's love of tools and gadgetry was Ambroise Paré, a sixteenth-century surgeon who designed surgical instruments, created prosthetic limbs from steel, invented steel corsets for scoliosis and steel boots for club feet, and introduced rudimentary surgical procedures, such as tying off large vessels during amputations.

Not only was Johns Hopkins's William Halsted a pivotal figure in the development of the practices that helped create modern surgery, but he also established the university's hospital as a leading center of surgical science. Several generations later, Johns Hopkins cardiac surgeon Vincent L. Gott observed and participated in some of the twentieth-century technological and surgical breakthroughs that save tens of thousands of lives today. At age 77, Gott—a tall, slender, distinguished-looking man with pewter-colored hair—no longer operates on patients but is still a professor of surgery.

After graduating from Yale Medical School, Gott trained from 1953 to 1960 at the University of Minnesota, where he had the good fortune to work under acclaimed heart surgeon C. Walton Lillehei, considered the father of open-heart surgery. Working with engineers such as Earl Bakken, the founder of the Medtronic corporation, Lillehei pioneered operations in the mid-1950s that brought some of the century's great biomedical engineering inventions to patients. The most notable was the development of the first battery-operated cardiac pacemaker with leads inserted directly into the heart. Lillehei—who performed open-heart surgery on forty-five children while keeping them alive by circulating their blood through their parents—also worked with Dr. Richard A. DeWall to devise a blood oxygenator. When patients' hearts were stopped during open-heart surgery, the oxygenator kept them alive by suffusing their blood with oxygen and recirculating it through the body. DeWall, whom Gott described as a "remarkable gadgeteer," played a major role in inventing the blood oxygenator. First employed in 1955, the DeWall-Lillehei blood oxygenator was widely used in open-heart surgery for the next twenty-five years. It was a precursor of the heart-lung pump now universally used to oxygenate patients' blood during heart bypass and other cardiopulmonary surgeries.

Gott went on to be the co-inventor of a heart valve coated with graphite and an anticlotting agent, and to develop new cardiac surgical techniques. Throughout his long career, he has retained his respect for the union of surgeons and engineers and is a major champion at Johns Hopkins of the novel, robotic techniques employed by his colleague David Yuh.

"Everything we're talking about—pacemakers, heart valves, blood oxygenators—was proposed by surgeons, but the surgeons did not have the wherewithal to do it," said Gott, who was director of cardiac surgery at Johns Hopkins for seventeen years. "The engineers were vital. Any device that has come along has always been a collaboration between surgeons and engineers."

Today, Gott's surgical colleagues at Johns Hopkins agree that biomedical engineering advances—superaccurate imaging, improved tools for robotic and minimally invasive surgery, and vastly improved machines to deliver anesthesia and monitor a patient's physiology during an operation—have led to far more effective and safer surgeries in the past two decades.

"All of this has made an incredible impact on our ability to assess patients and diagnose disease," said Dr. Julie Freischlag, 50, the first female director of the Department of Surgery at Johns Hopkins. "This has made operations safer, quicker, and less complicated. Now, imaging is everything. It helps you select the appropriate patients for surgery, and it limits how much time you have to be inside a patient. Thanks to imaging, you're rarely surprised anymore when you operate on a patient. Twenty years ago, we were sometimes very surprised."

A quarter century ago, when Freischlag was just beginning her surgical career, patients also died on the operating table more frequently. But today, with devices that can monitor a patient's heart through the esophagus, precisely measure blood gases and blood sugars, and deliver and monitor anesthesia far more effectively, operating room mortality has plummeted.

"I can't remember the last time someone died on the table here," said Freischlag, one of four female chiefs of surgery in the United States. "When I was an intern, it was far more common."

Young surgeons and surgical residents have wholeheartedly embraced the move toward robotic and high-tech surgery, said Freischlag. All now receive training at Johns Hopkins's Minimally Invasive Surgical Training Center, where they learn laparoscopic and robotic surgical techniques. But Freischlag considers it part of her mission to make sure that surgeons do not get so wrapped up in advanced imaging, robotics, and computers that they forget the human side of patient care.

"The young surgeons are extremely technologically savvy," said Freischlag, a vascular surgeon. "They love computers. They're terribly comfortable with robots. They're pretty virtual. The drawback is that we've lost the art of medicine somewhat. There is still a role for compassion. I still hold my patients' hands. I want young surgeons to know how to take a patient's history, to ask them, 'What's wrong with you? How do you feel? What do you want?' There's this whole piece of holding a patient's hand that we don't want to forget."

In the fields of heart and brain surgery, perhaps the most important development in recent decades is the arrival of real-time, detailed imaging in the operating room. Cardiac and neurological surgeons use highly detailed images—whether ultrasound, CT, or MR—both to plan surgeries and then to assess their work before they close up the patient. Dr. William A. Baumgartner, the chief of cardiac surgery at Johns Hopkins, said that surgeons performing heart valve replacement operations can obtain detailed, live images of the heart and its function through echocardiography (ultrasound) probes inserted in patients' throats.

"That technology has really allowed us to see continuously how the heart is doing," said Baumgartner, who frequently does coronary artery bypass procedures. "It sits there while you're operating. You can see the heart pump. You can see if the repair was good or not. If the repair isn't right, you do it over and get it right."

On the near horizon, said Baumgartner, is the development of rapid, extremely detailed CT and MR scans that will give cardiac surgeons a clear picture, in the operating room, of heart function and arterial blockage.

"It's phenomenal technology," said Baumgartner. "You can see all the arteries. It tells you what you need to know about blood flow in the heart."

In neurosurgery, ever more accurate CT and MR images already are being used to plan and carry out brain operations. One notable example is the use of such imaging to map out the vasculature of Siamese twins and plot the lengthy, complex separation surgery.

Russ Taylor, the director of Johns Hopkins's Center for Computer Integrated Surgical Systems and Technology, devised a system early in his career to help surgeons plan and execute complicated cranial/facial surgery using imaging and computer models. Now, Taylor and other scientists at the center collaborate with surgeons to develop systems in which engineers and surgeons precisely match the image of a patient with that person's anatomy, a process known as registering.

On a Johns Hopkins campus across town, in a lab called Urobotics, Dan Stoianovici—an associate professor of urology and mechanical engineering—has set up a workshop to further advance computer-assisted surgery. Using a life-size surgical dummy that breathes and has a heartbeat, Stoianovici and his team, in collaboration with Johns Hopkins surgeons, developed a system in which CT images are registered with a patient's anatomy. Using the CT image, a robot then guides a needle with an umbrella-shaped tip into the patient, enabling the surgeon to ablate, or burn, tumors in the liver, kidneys, lung, or spine using a high-frequency charge.

"The true potential of surgical robotics extends much beyond the da Vinci," said Stoianovici, a native of Romania. "To take full advantage of robotic surgery you need to integrate medical images. The real advantages are from the computer intelligence and imaging information the robot gets."

In an adjacent room, equipped with high-tech lathes and milling machines used to custom-make robots, Stoianovici showed me one of his works in progress. It was a robot, made entirely of nonmetallic parts, that could be used safely inside an MRI machine. Constructed of ceramics, acrylics, plastics, and glass and running on a pneumatic power system, lasers, and fiber optics, the blue and gray robotic arm hissed and rotated at Stoianovici's command. The robot, which would use live MR images for guidance, could make movements with a precision of 25 microns, about a third the width of a human hair.

"I'm very happy about this machine," Stoianovici said with a slight smile. "It's the only MRI compatible motor in the world."

In the lab of Johns Hopkins computer scientist Gregory Hager, researchers are investigating ways to employ finely calibrated robotic systems and imaging to target small vessels in diseased eyes or brains. Using the vasculature of chicken embryos as a training ground, the researchers are devising systems to automatically position tiny needles to deliver drugs, bust clots, or block growth in tiny vessels. One potential application is in the treatment of age-related macular degeneration, a common eye disease in the elderly in which an abnormal number of vessels grow behind the retina and leak blood and fluid, causing the loss of central vision. Collaborating with eye doctors at Johns Hopkins, Hager is investigating whether computer-assisted robotic surgery, working with detailed images of the eye's vasculature, could be used to block the rampant vessel growth that causes macular degeneration.

Dr. Michael R. Marohn, a Johns Hopkins gastrointestinal surgeon who collaborates with Hager, said he envisions a day when surgeons will view detailed, three-dimensional images transposed on a screen along with live pictures of a patient's insides. The two images will be precisely matched, or registered, allowing the surgeon to command the robot to move to a spot inside the body that corresponds to the tumor or anomaly on the image. The surgeon can then operate with the assistance of the robot. By registering images with the patient's anatomy, the robot could be programmed to be "locked out" of certain areas, preventing it, for example, from getting near a major vessel like the vena cava.

"When you start thinking where this could go, it gets pretty exciting," said Marohn, who has performed about 200 surgeries with the da Vinci robot. "I think computer-assisted surgery will really change how we do things, and when you pull in imaging it gets really promising. You could have the robot do some or all of the surgery. The precision of robotic registration with images is not good enough now, but it's getting there. What we're trying to do is build that collaboration with the engineering school more and more. The lines among surgeons, engineers, and the imaging people are starting to be blurred, and that's going to be better for the patients."

Marohn also is intrigued by the potential of long-distance surgery, one of the initial motivations in creating the da Vinci system. The high point in that realm came on September 7, 2001, when a team of surgeons at Mt. Sinai Hospital in New York City took fifty-four minutes to remove the gall bladder of a patient in Strasbourg, France. The commands were transmitted from a Zeus robotic system in New York to a Zeus system in Strasbourg using a fiber-optic cable. "Why not be able to remotely project expertise?" said Marohn, who was a surgeon in the U.S. Air Force before coming to Johns Hopkins.

Hager, Marohn, and others are also interested in coupling the da

Vinci robot and computer programs to develop simulators—much like flight simulators—to be used in surgical training.

"We can take the motion tracer from the da Vinci and trace the surgical gestures of a leading surgeon," said Hager. "In suturing, for example, we can observe a good surgeon and parse that into suturing steps. You can have a surgeon in training and you can evaluate how they're doing. How did they deviate from the gestures of a leading surgeon? We're talking about virtual training and mentoring, using computers to learn about surgery and correct what you do. In almost every other discipline you have some notion of quantitative assessment."

Johns Hopkins mechanical engineer Allison M. Okamura believes that working on surgical simulators will become a standard aspect of surgical training, in part because of research she and others are doing in the field of haptics. "Haptics" involves the sense of touch, and Okamura, along with other academic and industrial researchers nationwide, is trying to figure out how to give surgeons the same fine, tactile sensations using a robot or a simulator that they enjoy when performing surgery with their own hands. At present, the da Vinci system provides surgeons such as Yuh no sense of the force they are applying when making an incision, screwing a pacemaker lead into cardiac muscle, suturing a wound, or tying a surgical knot. Instead, Yuh and his colleagues rely primarily on observing the indentations that their actions make on tissue.

"You can't really feel anything, and conceivably you could do a lot of damage working with an organ like the heart," said Yuh. "General surgeons say this lack of feeling hasn't bothered them as much. They work with tissue, like bowel or muscle, that is more forgiving. But in cardiac surgery we're working with arteries so thin you can see through them or with vessels so hardened with plaque that they can crack. Heart tissue is very hard to work with, and Allison is collaborating with us because of the nature of the tissue we deal with."

Yuh said that biomedical engineers, surgeons, and companies like Intuitive Surgical, which manufactures the da Vinci, all realize the importance of developing tactile feedback systems. Although some surgeons have performed cardiac artery bypass surgeries on a trial basis with the da Vinci robot, Yuh believes that the operation is not "reproducibly excellent," in part because of the lack of a sense of touch needed in suturing coronary artery grafts.

"The consequences of doing a bad job are tremendous in bypass surgery, and you want to get it right the first time," said Yuh. "I don't doubt that bypass surgeries will be done that way someday. We've come a long way in understanding how important haptics is and how difficult it is to build it into a robotic instrument."

The problem, said Okamura, is a classic engineering challenge of "signals and systems," which in this case means picking up a signal from the robot arm and transmitting it via cables and computers to the hand controls of the surgeon. The surgeon's gestures must then be transmitted back to the arm through the same pipeline. It sounds simple, but Okamura said there are numerous obstacles, including time delays and the difficulty of creating gauges and sensors that mimic the fine tactile system of the human hand. In addition, said Okamura, "We're trying to figure out how to do all this cheaply and with small instruments."

For now, the solution that Okamura and her graduate students are focusing on is a system that, using a bar graph, would display the force being applied by the surgeon and the resistance he or she is encountering. That graph, which could resemble the digital volume controls seen on televisions or computers, would be placed in the surgeon's field of vision as he or she looks through the eyepieces on the robot.

"This may not be as good as giving feedback directly to the surgeon's hand," said Okamura, "but the visual display system is much farther along and is more promising in the short run. We think it's a practical way to integrate force feedback into the robot."

In Okamura's lab, master's student Carol Reiley showed me some prototypes of the visual system. In one, she manipulated the 18-inch da Vinci arm, and a green bar graph on a computer screen expanded or contracted based on the intensity of her squeeze. In another system, a green circle shrank or enlarged depending on the force applied. Similar visual cues could be transmitted to surgeons based on the resistance of the tissue they suture or cut. Indeed, other students in Okamura's lab are involved in using a robot to cut real tissue. Their aim is to develop scales of resistance based on the kind of tissue being sliced or sutured.

"If robotic surgery is going to become widespread, you're going to have to have that tactile feedback," said Yuh. "Haptic feedback will make operations safer and will speed them up. A lot of time I spend now on the da Vinci is making sure I'm not putting too much or too little tension on the sutures. That takes more time. Surgery is a series of steps, and in heart surgery the faster the surgery, the better. Time does matter. You're on the clock."

Surgery is generally a conservative field, for the obvious reason that when wielding life or death power over a patient a surgeon is likely to stick to tried and true techniques. The field was initially skeptical of both laparoscopic and robotic surgery, and many surgeons "went in kicking and screaming" as these new surgical techniques began to spread, said Louis R. Kavoussi, professor of urologic surgery at Johns Hopkins. (Laparoscopy was developed over the course of the twentieth century by a series of surgeons who experimented with introducing needles and surgical instruments into the abdominal cavity.) But after people began hearing about the wonders of laparoscopic surgery in the late 1980s, particularly for gall bladder removal, "the public drove the demand" and surgeons followed, said Kavoussi. Today, 95 percent of the 700,000 gall bladder removal surgeries performed annually in the United States are done laparoscopically, as people prefer the small scars and faster recovery times of minimally invasive operations.

One Johns Hopkins physician, Anthony N. Kalloo—the director of the Division of Gastroenterology and Hepatology—is pushing surgery to new levels. He is now experimenting in pigs with a new technique, known as transgastric surgery, that involves placing an endoscope down the throat and into the stomach and then cutting through the stomach wall and operating inside the abdominal cavity. Traditional endoscopic surgery owes a great deal to British optical physicist Harold Hopkins, who in 1957 perfected the technique of transmitting light and images through glass fibers inside a flexible tube, thus creating the fiber-optic endoscope.

To date, Kalloo and his associates have used this technique to tie the fallopian tubes of pigs, repair hernias, and remove spleens by cutting them out and pulling them through the stomach and the throat. The method also could be used for gall bladder surgery. The stomach wall is highly contractile and with a few staples heals completely, rapidly, and relatively painlessly, said Kalloo.

"What I've done is take the concept of minimally invasive surgery one step further and avoid an external incision altogether," said Kalloo. "This may be a perfect technique for obese patients because one of the challenges of operating on obese patients is cutting through the thick abdominal wall."

Just as many patients have become strong supporters of laparoscopic surgery, robotic surgery is expected to gain wider acceptance as its benefits become known. Indeed, despite the lack of tactile feedback, surgeons at Johns Hopkins and elsewhere say that robotic systems like the da Vinci are increasingly popular with surgeons and the public.

"This is a wristed instrument with a lot of flexibility," said Dr. Mark A. Talamini, a gastrointestinal surgeon and director of Minimally Invasive Surgery at the Johns Hopkins University School of Medicine. "You're in virtual reality in the corner of the operating room, and it's like you're walking around inside the abdomen. The 3-D vision can be even better than with your own eyes. The most dramatic development in the OR recently has been robotics. It's a fascinating story, although the jury is still out."

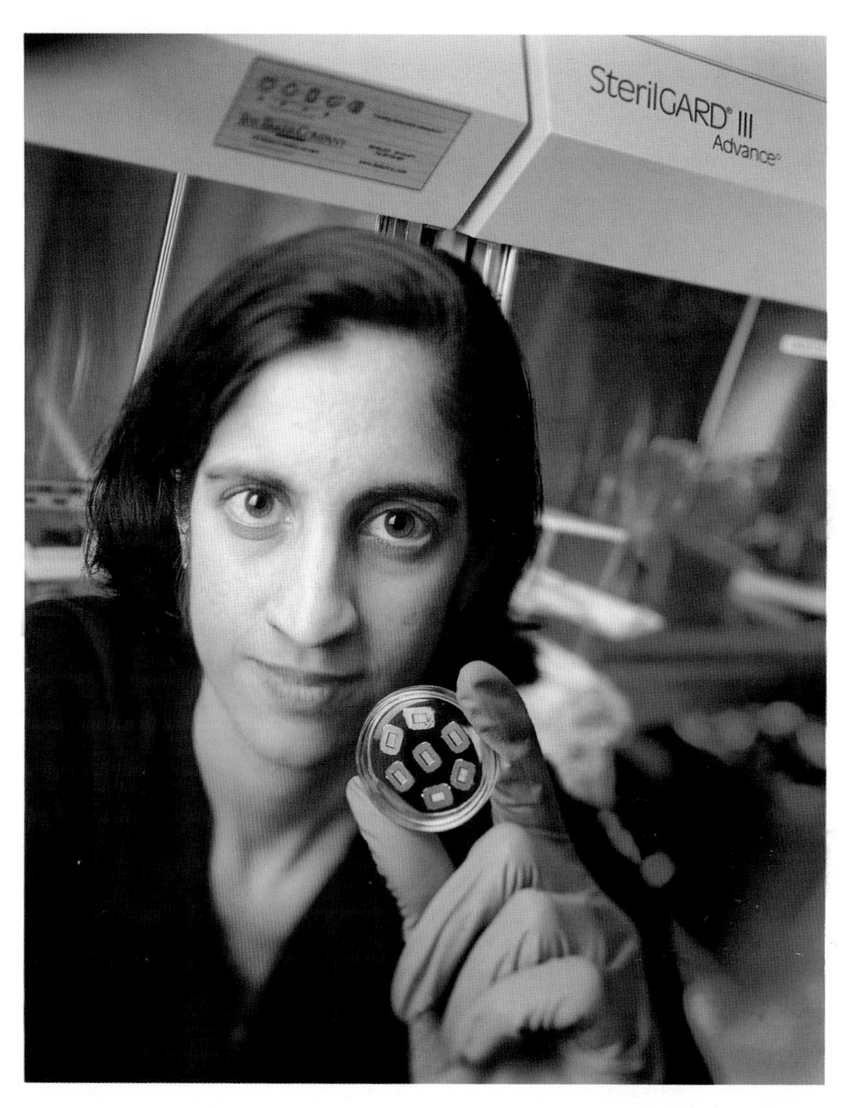

Tejal Desai is part of a new generation of researchers that has focused on micro applications of biomedical engineering. She is displaying the fruits of MEMS technology (micro-electrical-mechanical systems), in which small chips are being investigated as implantable replacements for diseased organs such as the pancreas. Photograph by Peter Howard

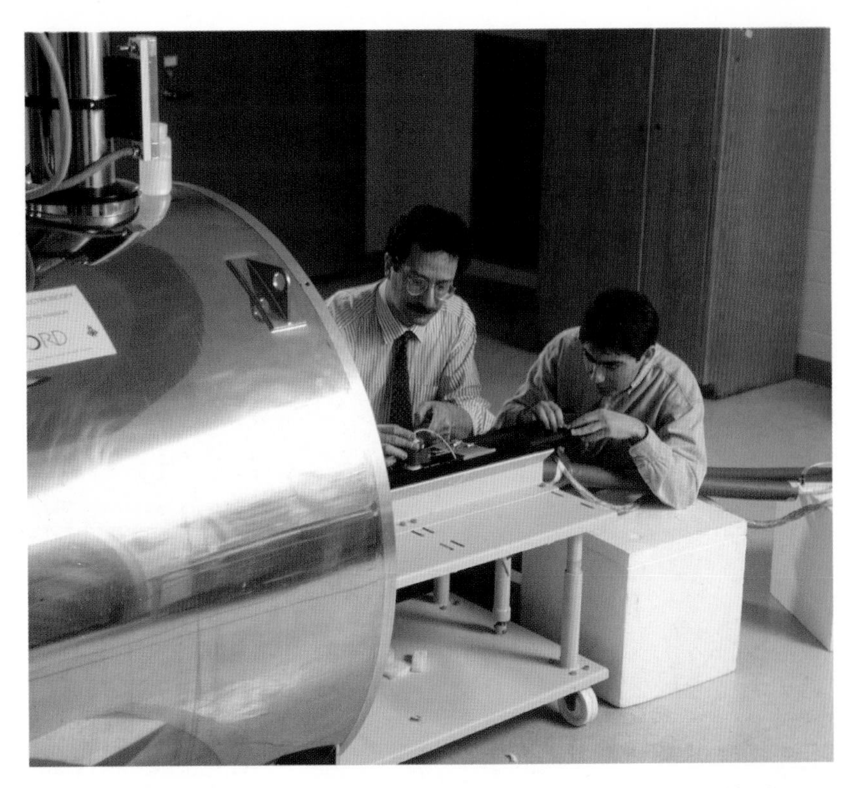

Georgia Tech researcher Athanassios Sambanis is attempting to develop an artificial pancreas to aid people with severe diabetes. Photograph by Jack Kearse

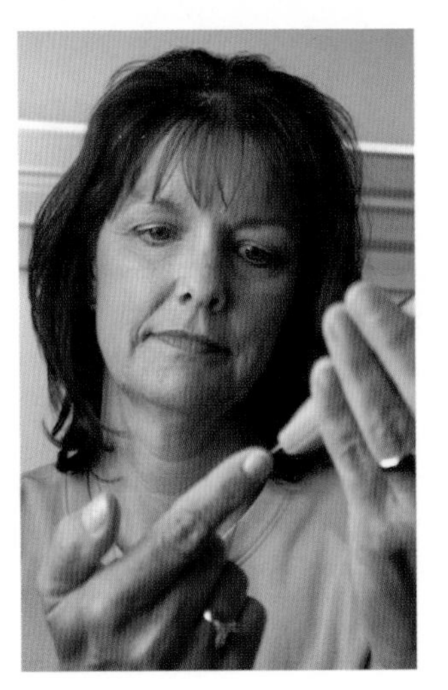

Laura Cochran of Columbus, Georgia, was the recipient of transplanted pancreatic cells, an operation that rid her of devastating Type 1 diabetes, although she periodically checks her blood sugar levels. The treatment offers a hint of possible treatments that may one day emerge from the field of tissue engineering. Photograph by Ken Hawkins

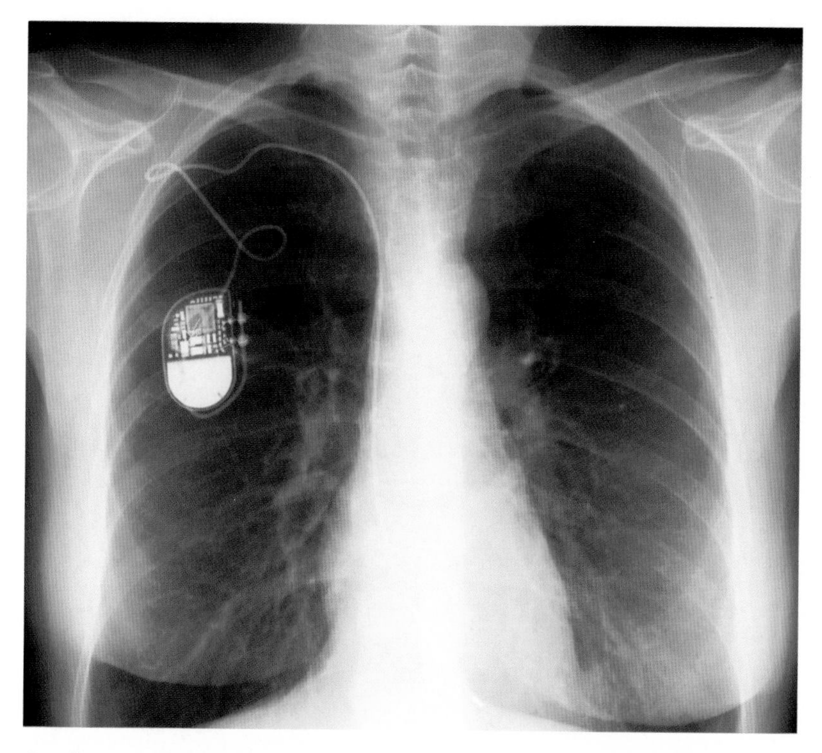

Cardiac pacemakers, implanted in one million people worldwide every year, are widely considered to be one of biomedical engineering's greatest inventions. Photograph courtesy of Getty Images

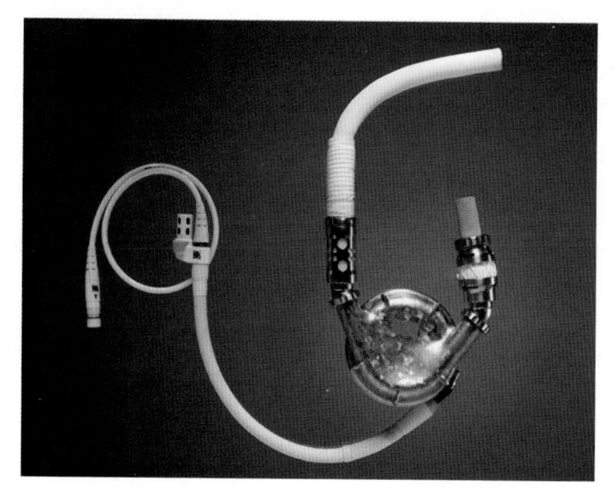

The HeartMate left ventricular assist device (LVAD) took more than two decades to develop. Image courtesy of Thoratec Corporation

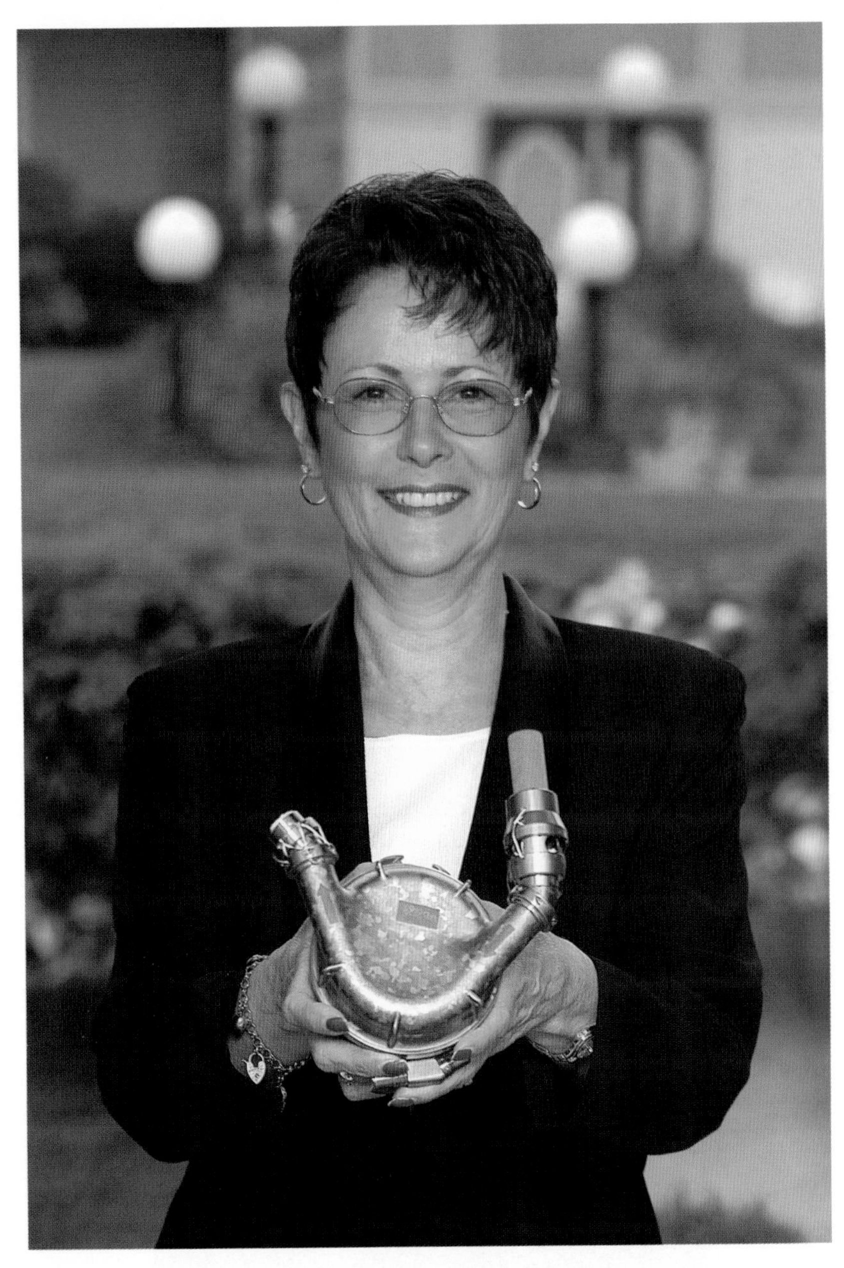

Roxanne Emswiler of Harrisonburg, Virginia, was stricken with a life-threatening heart condition and placed on a list to receive a heart transplant. She was kept alive with a left ventricular assist device, which assumes the pumping function of the crucial left ventricle, until her successful transplant surgery. Photograph by William K. Geiger

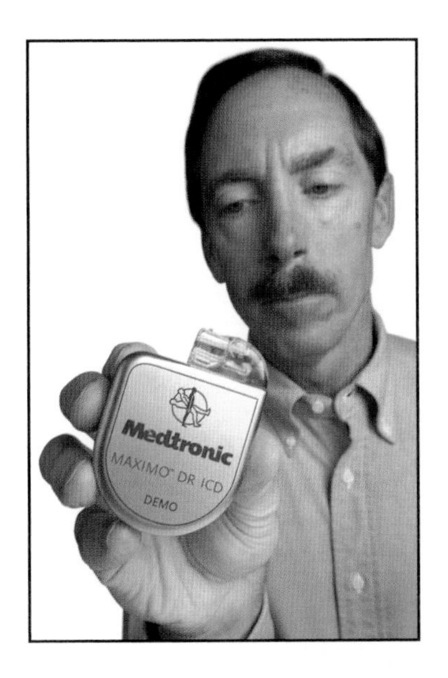

Jay Joyce of Cincinnati has a rare heart condition that required him to receive an implantable defibrillator, which interrupts the rapid, chaotic, and potentially fatal beating of the heart, known as ventricular fibrillation. Photograph by Christopher Navin

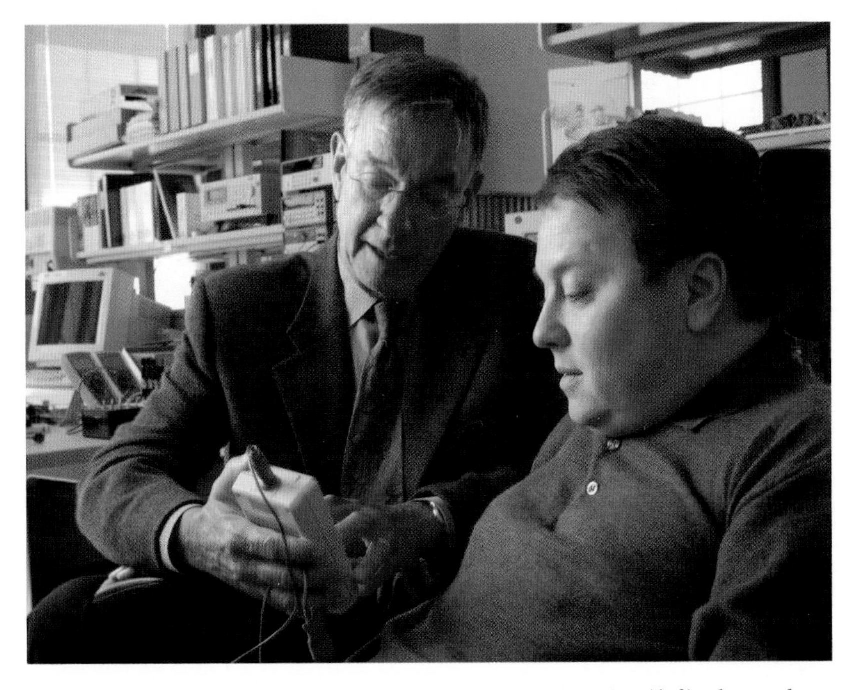

J. Thomas Mortimer of Case Western Reserve University (*left*), shown here with patient Laszlo Nagy. Mortimer was one of the pioneers of implanting electrodes in spinal cord injury patients to restore movement and enable them to breathe. Photograph by Ken Hawkins

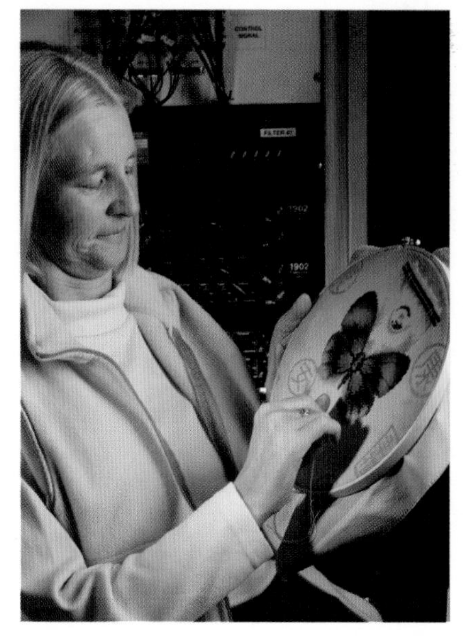

Annette Coker, paralyzed from the chest down in an automobile accident, has regained much of the use of her hands and arms thanks to implanted electrodes that stimulate her muscles. Her device was specially outfitted so she could resume a favorite pastime, needlepoint. Photograph by Ken Hawkins

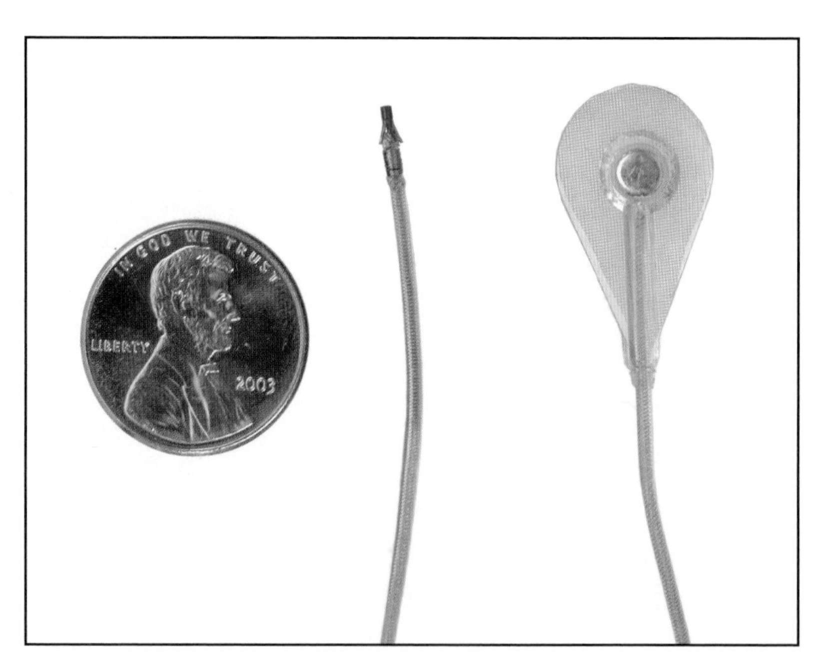

Implantable electrodes can be placed in or on the muscles of a paralyzed person to restore partial use. The two electrodes shown here are small enough that they can be placed into or on a variety of muscles. Photograph courtesy of Cleveland FES Center

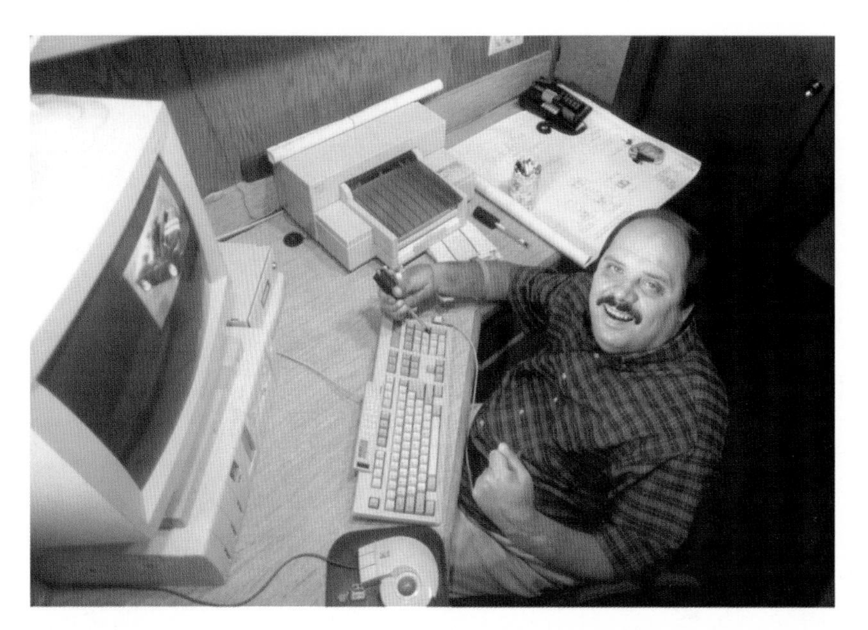

Quadriplegic Jim Jatich was the first patient at Case Western Reserve University to receive a network of implanted electrodes in his arms. Case and its partners are pioneers in so-called functional electrical stimulation (FES). Photograph courtesy of Cleveland FES Center

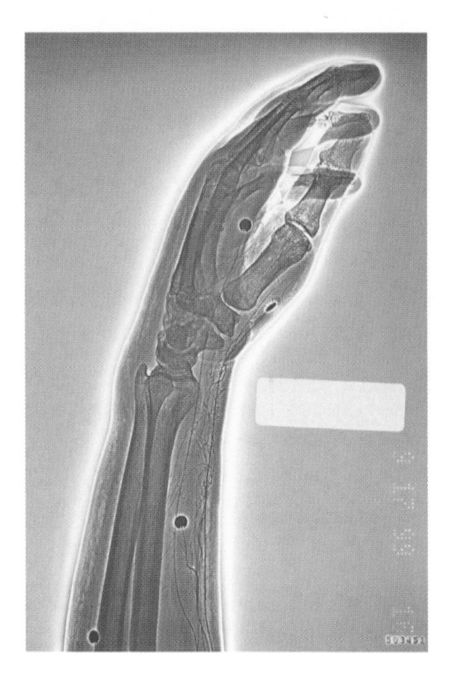

An X-ray image reveals the electrodes implanted in Jim Jatich's arm and hand. Photograph by P. Hunter Peckham

What's Happening in the Brain? Medical imaging technology makes it possible to see brain structure and function with remarkable clarity. These technologies aid in understanding the healthy brain and in diagnosing illness.

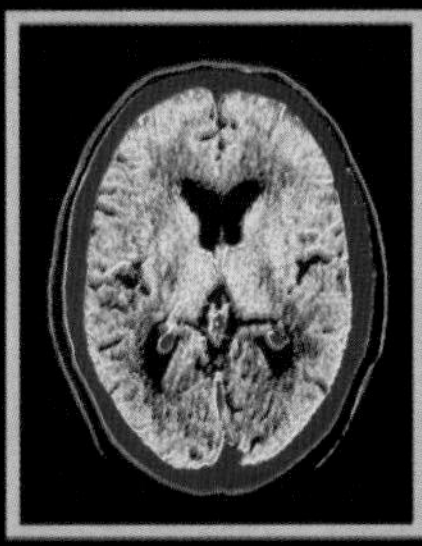

CT Scan
A CT (computerized tomography) scan combines X-rays with computer technology to produce a precise image of a cross section of the brain. It is used to detect tumors, blood clots, birth defects, and certain kinds of brain damage.

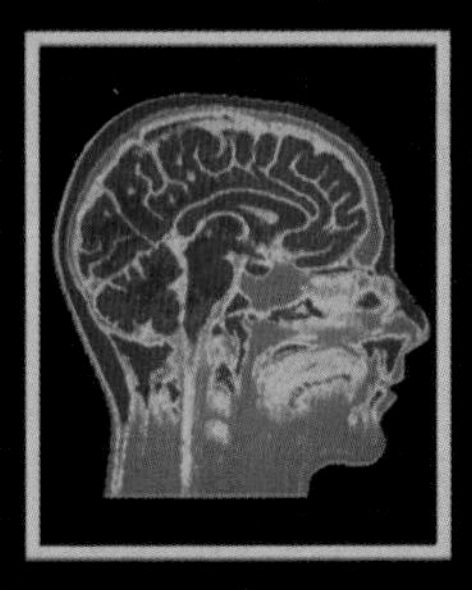

MRI
MRI (magnetic resonance imaging) reveals blood vessels, brain, spinal cord, and other types of soft tissue. It uses a strong but harmless magnetic field to produce detailed cross-section images that can show abnormalities and brain diseases.

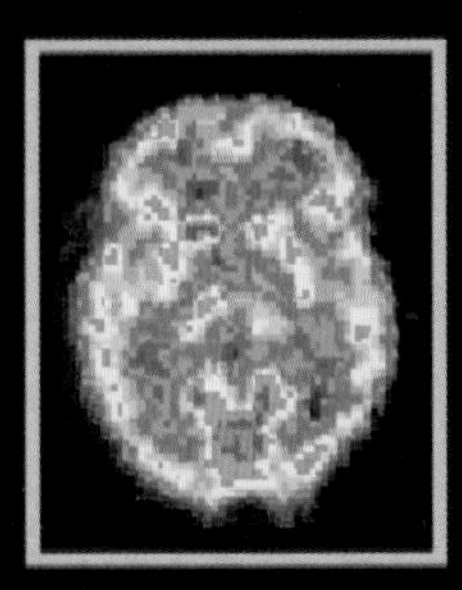

PET Scan
A PET (positron emission tomography) scan is a picture of the brain at work. When the brain works, it uses glucose. A PET scan shows glucose levels in the brain. Shades of red and yellow indicate the most active regions. Areas that are green and blue are less active.

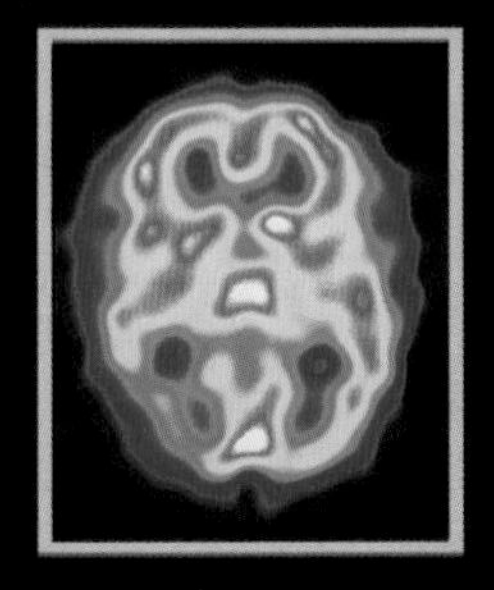

SPECT
For single-photon emission computerized tomography, the patient ingests a small amount of radioactive tracer that emits photons of energy. A photon detector rotates around the target area, capturing images that are combined in a computer to make a three-dimensional picture.

Few realms of biomedical engineering have had as much impact as imaging, which has changed the face of medicine. Shown here are different imaging techniques used in analyzing how a patient's brain is functioning. Photographs courtesy of MSK Partners

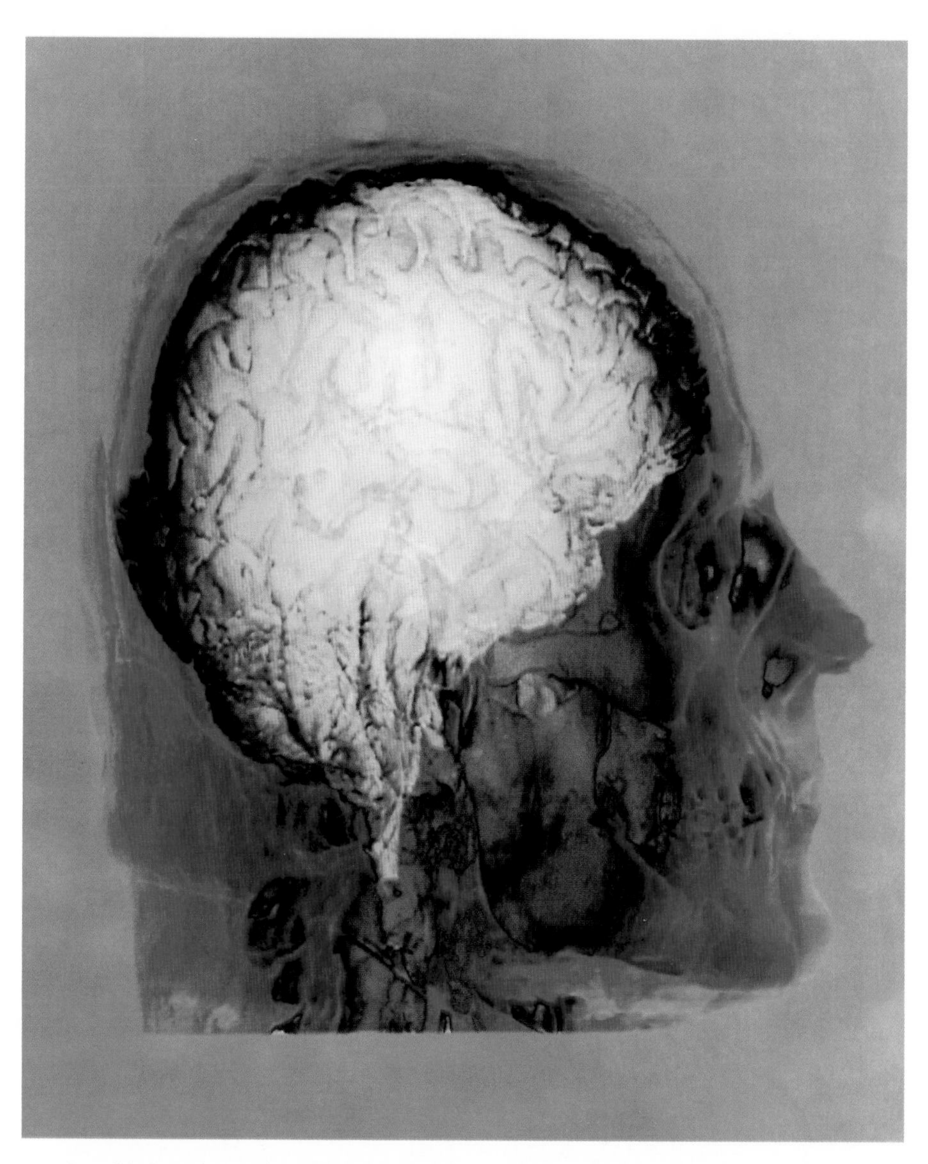

Combining three-dimensional computerized tomography (CT) and magnetic resonance (MR) imaging allows this brain to be mapped out in advance of surgery. Photograph courtesy of Photo Researchers

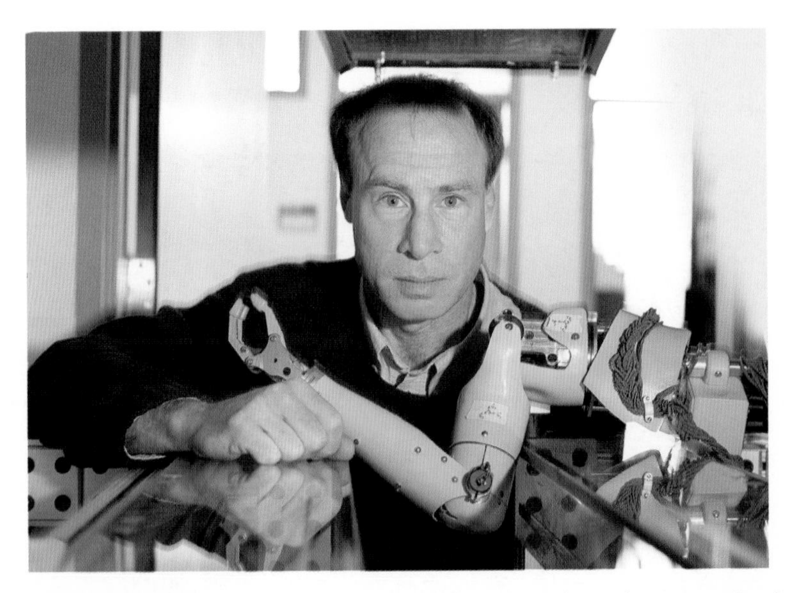

Andrew Schwartz of the University of Pittsburgh with a robotic arm he developed to test the ability of monkeys to move the arm using only thoughts. Photograph by Peter Howard

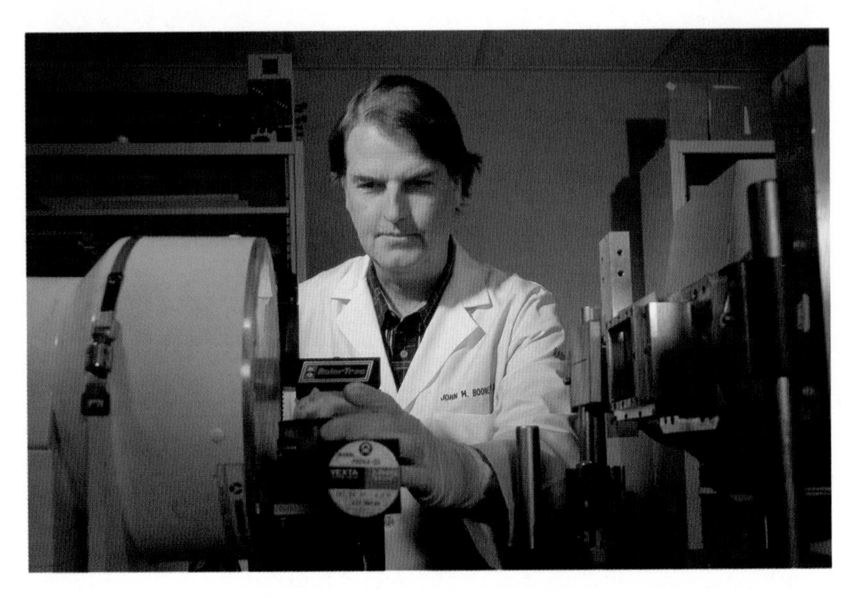

John Boone of the University of California, Davis, Cancer Center has invented a new CT (computerized tomography) scan for the breast that can detect tumors at a significantly earlier stage than conventional mammography. Photograph courtesy of The Regents of the University of California

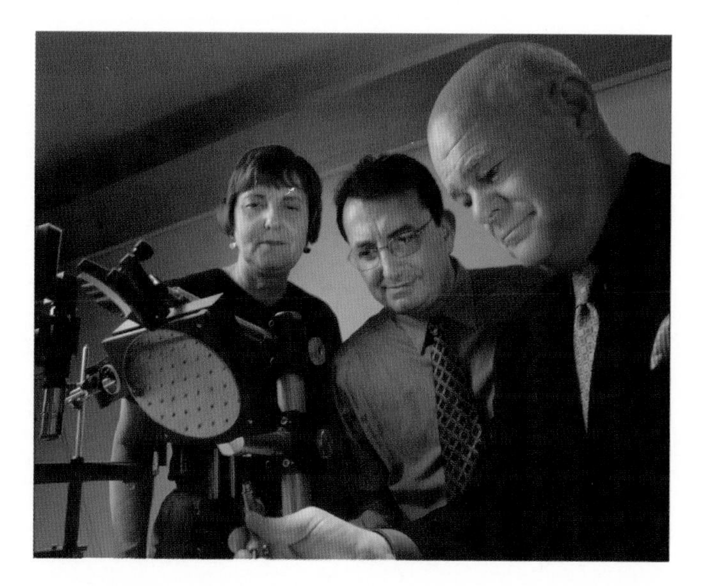

Ralph deVere White (*right*), the director of the University of California, Davis, Cancer Center, which is investigating ways of imaging and treating tumors with highly targeted molecular agents. Photograph courtesy of The Regents of the University of California

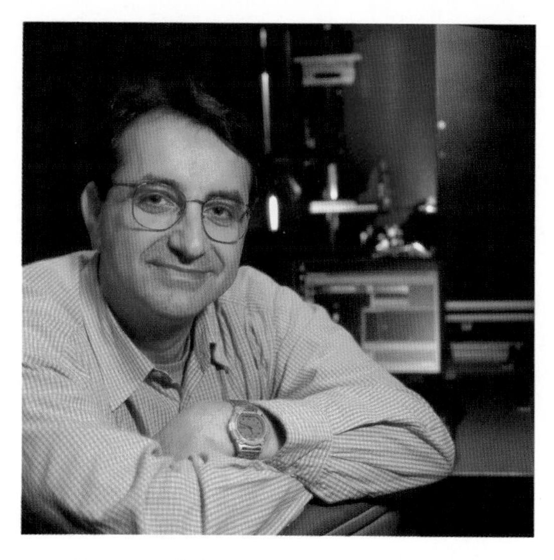

Researcher Stavros Demos of the University of California, Davis, Cancer Center has developed a novel use of different kinds of light to detect cancerous lesions in the bladder. Photograph courtesy of The Regents of the University of California

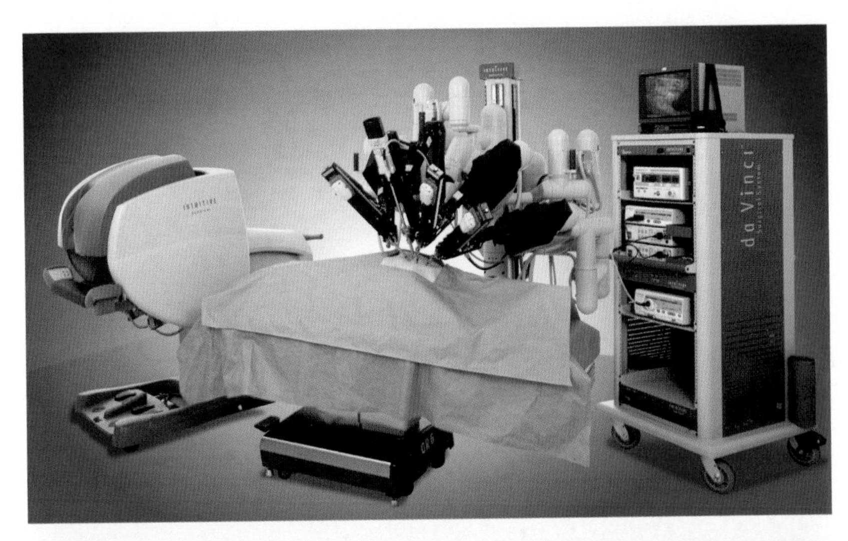

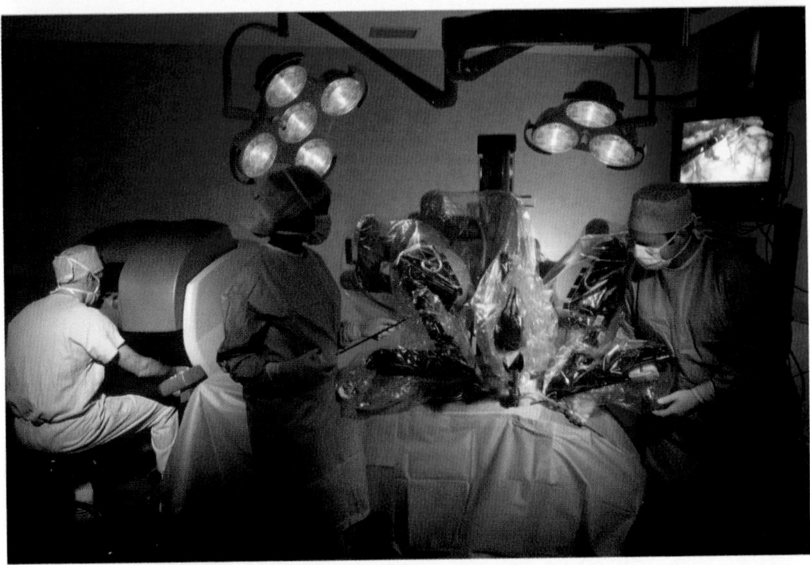

The da Vinci robotic surgery system enables surgeons to perform certain operations less invasively and more effectively than traditional surgery. The da Vinci is used for a number of operations, including heart valve repair. The somewhat daunting system, shown in its entirety at top, is making its way into more and more operating theaters (*bottom*). Images courtesy of Intuitive Surgical, Inc. © 2005

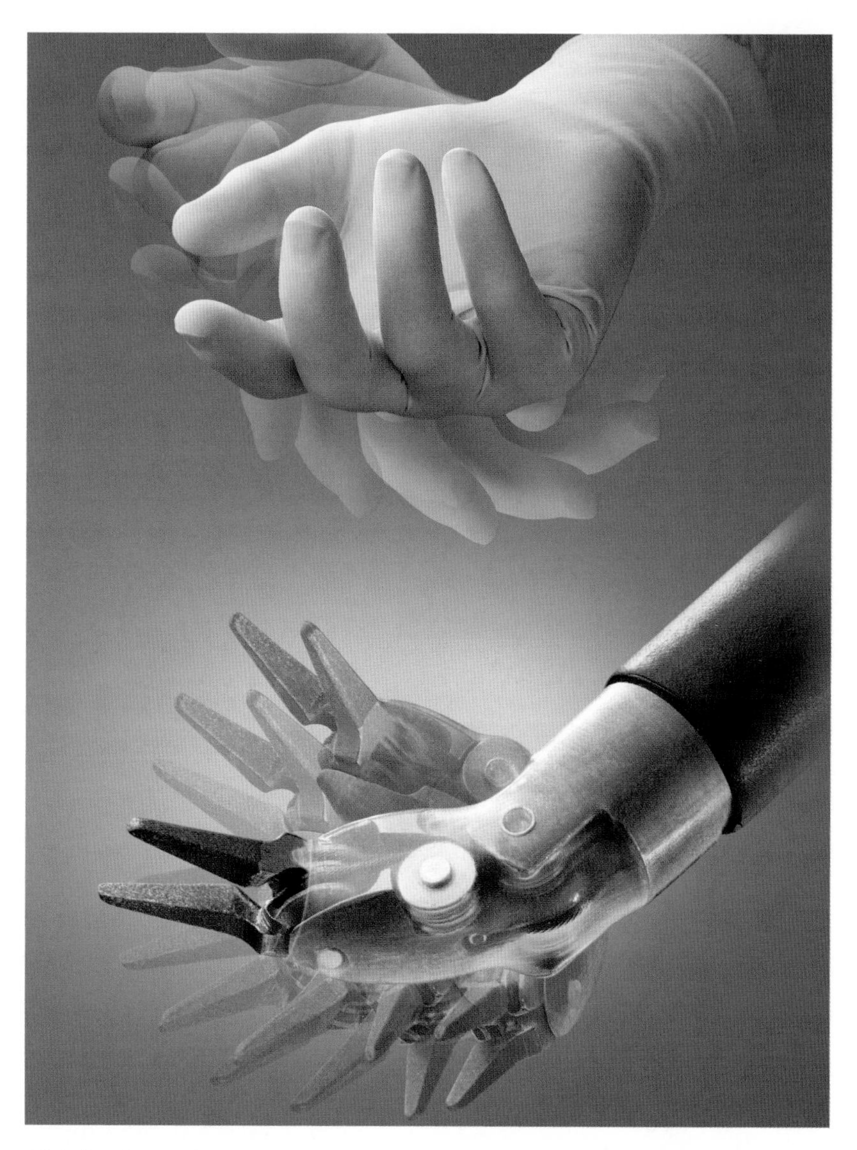

The da Vinci robotic arm as compared with a surgeon's hand. Image courtesy of Intuitive Surgical, Inc. © 2005

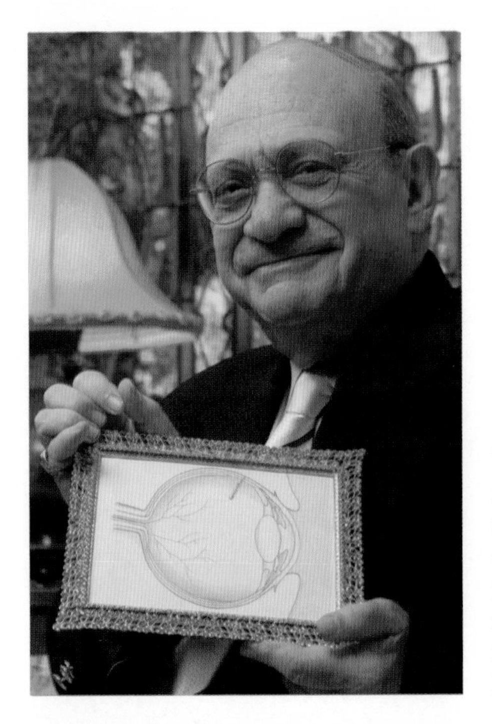

Theodore Hersh, himself a medical doctor, has retinitis pigmentosa, a retinal disease that eventually causes blindness. He reported significant improvement in his sight with the Neurotech device. Photograph by Ken Hawkins

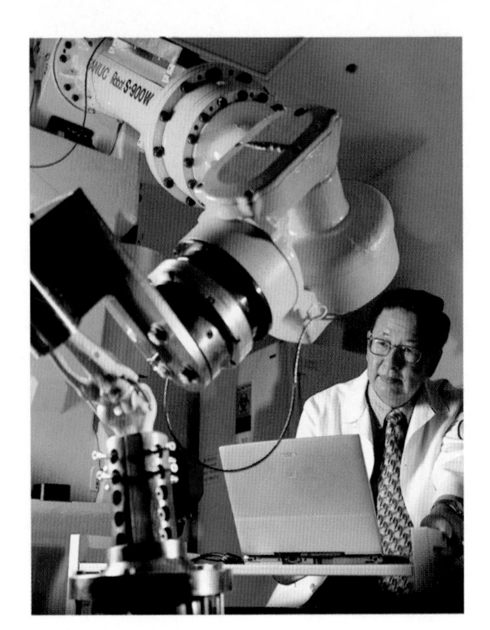

Savio L.-Y. Woo uses robots to study the forces applied on human joints. The robot moves actual bones (*foreground*) to duplicate injurious movements. Photograph by Peter Howard

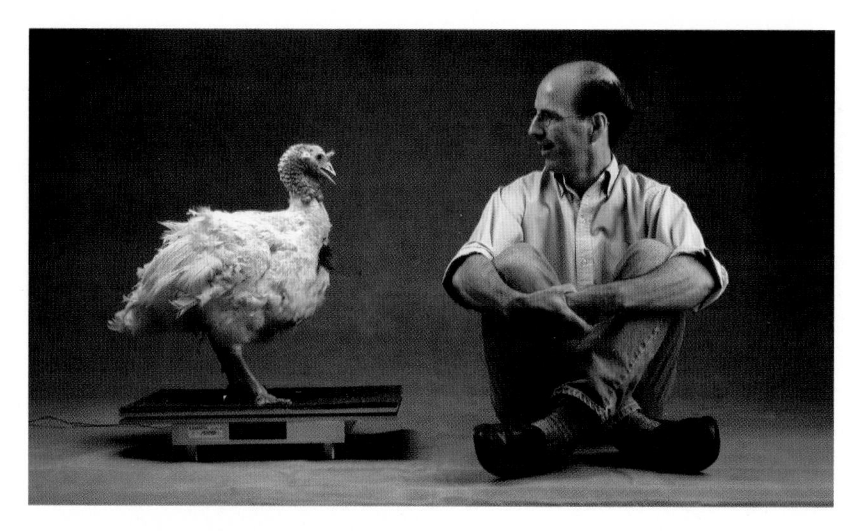

Experimenting first with turkeys and then with humans, Clinton Rubin of the State University of New York at Stony Brook discovered that bone loss associated with osteoporosis could be significantly reduced by briefly standing on a gently vibrating platform every day. Photograph by Cary Wolinsky / IPN / Aurora

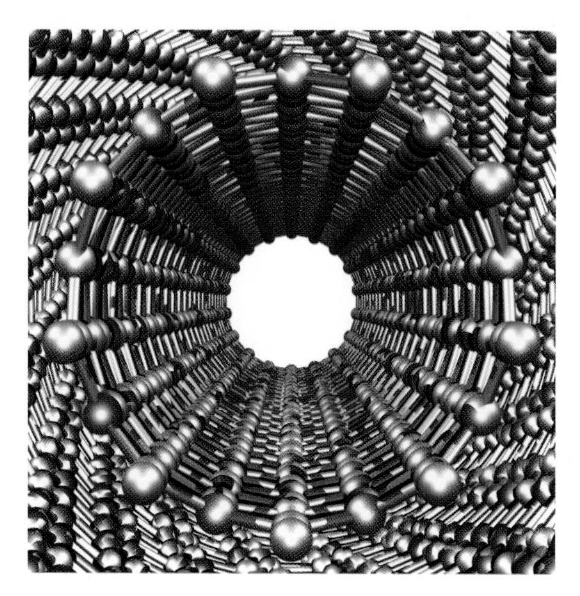

This computer-generated image of a double-walled nanotube shows a view through the length of the inner barrel. Nano, meaning "one-billionth," is a size that may provide biomedical engineers access to the smallest human structures. Courtesy of Chris Ewels

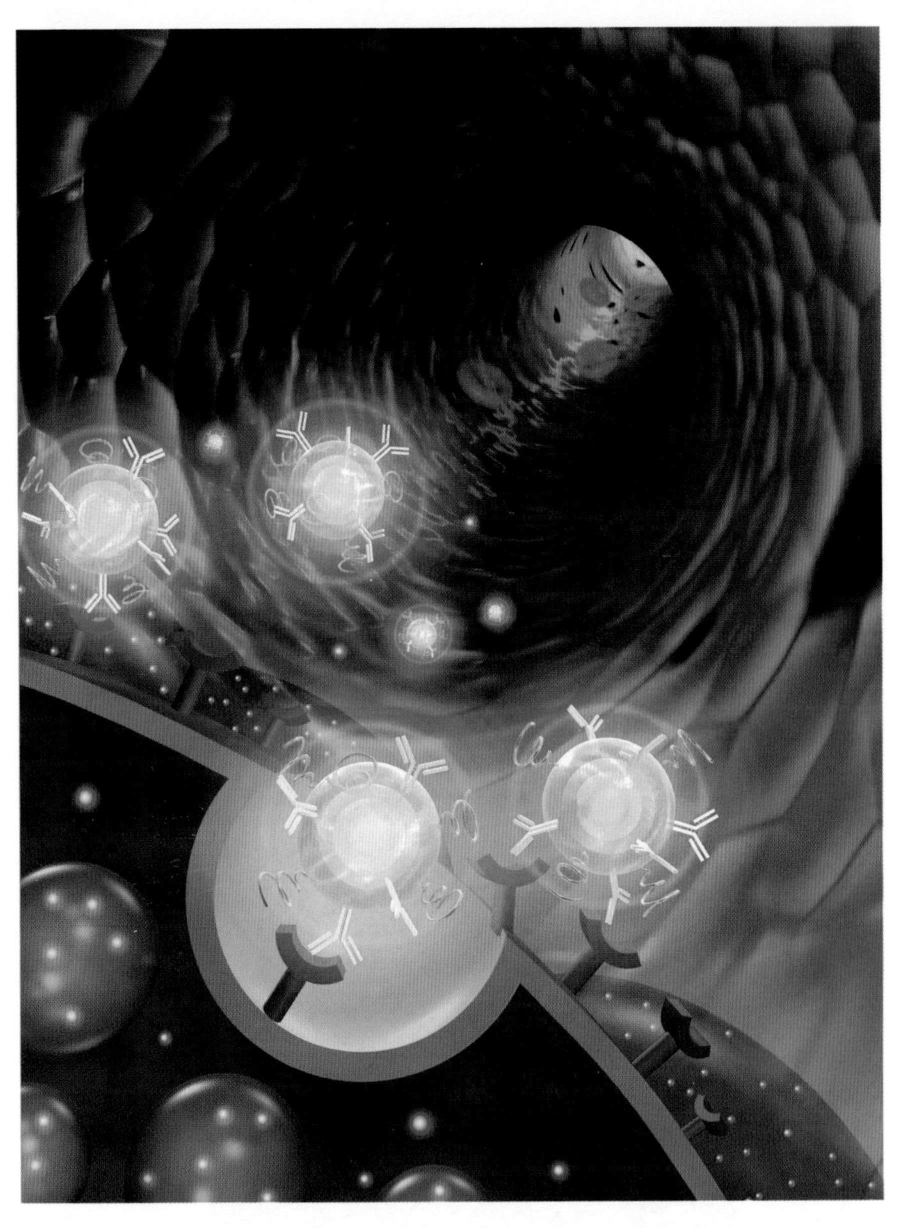

Tiny crystals, known as "quantum dots," are being explored as treatments for various maladies. This depiction of quantum dots shows them traveling inside a blood vessel as they seek out tumor cells. Courtesy of Nature Publishing Group, © Biatrix

CHAPTER 10

Bones

In Pittsburgh, along the banks of the Monongahela River, the giant steel mills that once dominated the city's landscape are giving way to low-slung, modern glass buildings that contain the offices and labs of the health care and high-tech industry. Not far from the river, on a warm September morning in 2004, orthopedic surgeon Patrick J. McMahon was in a satellite hospital of the University of Pittsburgh Medical Center, scrubbing up for a surgery that has come to symbolize the achievements of biomedical engineering and orthopedics. An assistant professor of orthopedic surgery at the university, McMahon was preparing to replace a patient's joint, in this case the left shoulder of 62-year-old Shirley A. Thompson. For several years, Thompson had been suffering from osteoarthritis, a degenerative disease in which the cartilage that cushions joints breaks down, causing pain and immobility as bone rubs against bone.

"It had gotten to the point where I couldn't raise my arm above my waist," Thompson, who works as an admissions clerk in a hospital emergency room, said after the operation. "I was in real bad shape. I couldn't hold my grandchildren. I couldn't lie on that side and couldn't sleep. I would come home from work and cry my pain was so bad. It was terrible."

In the operating room, McMahon—an outgoing, silver-haired man in his mid-forties—showed me an X-ray image of Thompson's shoulder joint. He pointed out how the diseased cartilage had left no gap between the humeral bone of the upper arm and the shoulder socket.

"You see the bones are flat together," said McMahon. "That's bone on bone, and when you've got bone on bone, it's only a question of how much pain you can take and how long you can take it. No medical treatment has had an impact on people with severe osteoarthritis or rheumatoid arthritis like total joint replacement."

A shoulder and elbow specialist who does 50 shoulder replacement surgeries a year—a total of 50,000 such operations are performed annually in the United States—McMahon was dressed in the usual blue-green surgical gown. But he also wore a clear plastic helmet, a sign that this surgery, like other joint replacement operations, would involve some heavy-duty labor and spattering of blood and tissue.

Thompson was covered by sterile surgical paper, with only her shoulder exposed. She was about to receive the Global Advantage Shoulder Arthroplasty System, an artificial joint from Du Puy Orthopedics, a division of Johnson & Johnson. It consisted of a titanium humeral prosthesis that would be inserted inside her bone. The exterior of the prosthesis was etched with a special filigree to encourage the ingrowth of Thompson's bone. The prosthesis was capped with a durable chrome and cobalt head that would be fitted into a high-grade-plastic socket. That socket, in turn, would be drilled and glued into Thompson's defective socket, which had been eroded by the arthritis and years of abrasion from the humeral bone. The weak link in the artificial joint, McMahon informed me, has long been the plastic socket, but he said that Du Puy had made significant strides recently in devising plastics that would last for many years.

Assisted by junior surgeon Leslie Beasley, McMahon—who also serves as assistant physician for the University of Pittsburgh football team—spent the next couple of hours carrying out what, at times, looked more like a home improvement project than an operation. He and Beasley reamed, ground, hammered, chiseled, and glued, and in the end Thompson, who has three children and six grandchildren, wound up with a new, snug-fitting shoulder that would put an end to her pain and immobility. As Beasley and a surgical resident put the finishing touches on the surgery in early afternoon, McMahon stepped away from the operating table and said, "There was a time when these prostheses broke. But now we've reached the point where this is about as good as it gets. So much of what we're able to do in orthopedics is the result of really good biomechanical research."

With the surgery completed, Thompson became one of more than 600,000 Americans who each year receive new hips, knees, shoulders, elbows, and ankles, enabling them to overcome crippling arthritis and joint injuries. Her operation came more than forty years after the first total joint replacement procedures were invented and carried out by English surgeon Sir John Charnley, who performed a series of hip replacements in the late 1950s and early 1960s.

"I'm doing really well," Thompson said seven months after the surgery. "I can lift my arm above my head and lie on my left side. On a scale of one to ten I would say the pain is now a one. It was just an excellent operation." She is already contemplating having McMahon do the same operation on her right shoulder, which has also become afflicted with osteoarthritis.

Joining McMahon in the operating room was David Stanek, a representative from Du Puy Orthopedics. Both men agreed that the next major development in joint replacement surgery would be what numerous investigators at Johns Hopkins and other universities are working on: computer-assisted surgery. With the aid of computers and possibly robots, surgeons will make ever smaller incisions, which could lead to smaller artificial joints. Much farther into the future, McMahon said that tissue engineering and, ultimately, molecular and genetic therapies may either halt the degenerative processes that ruin joints or provide ways of naturally regrowing cartilage.

"We look to the day when we don't have to do joint replacement," said McMahon.

If and when that day comes, it will represent the latest step in a long, fruitful collaboration between orthopedic surgeons and biomedical engineers. This partnership has brought immense benefits to millions of people worldwide who have received artificial joints. At the University of Pittsburgh, McMahon works closely with biomedical engineer Savio L.-Y. Woo, director of the Musculoskeletal Research Center. Engineers and physicians at the center are using a wide variety of methods—from robotic testing to cellular and molecular research—to understand the pathology of joints, ligaments, and tendons and how to repair them.

At the University of California, San Diego, and at Pitt—where he arrived in 1990—Woo has spent his career studying how ligaments, tendons, and other skeletal tissues respond to various influences. After doing numerous rabbit experiments in the late 1970s, he became one of the earliest proponents of what is now standard practice in orthopedics: encouraging controlled motion in a joint after an operation, rather than immobilizing the limb in a cast, which had the effect of freezing the joint and damaging cartilage, making recovery far more arduous.

"It was like spot welding the joints," said Woo. "Fortunately today after joint operations you don't see casts anymore. When I first got into orthopedics, you could see loads and loads of people putting on casts."

Woo's research also led to another discovery: that a vital ligament inside the knee—the medial collateral ligament, or MCL—could heal itself without surgery. The reason was that, unlike the anterior cruciate ligament (ACL), the MCL is encased in soft tissue and blood and undergoes a natural healing process after injury. (Damaged MCLs, however, often do not recover 100 percent.) Such discoveries have convinced Woo that the best treatments in orthopedics enlist the body to do as much work as possible.

"I want the body to do its thing because I just don't think we can do better than the body," said Woo, who is 63.

The practical bent of Woo's research center was on display during the week I visited the Musculoskeletal Research Center. There, on most days, teams of biomedical engineers and physicians were testing human cadaver shoulders and knees with a robot, part of an effort to discover the best surgical techniques to repair various injuries. On one occasion, the research team was replicating the damage done to the rounded top of the upper arm, or humeral, bone during shoulder dislocation. A humeral bone was cemented into a metal base, while the shoulder blade and socket were attached to the arm of a 7-foot robot. With sensors implanted in the shoulder and a camera recording the action, the robot repeatedly rotated the shoulder blade until the arm came out of its socket, an event that can fracture or chip the top end of the humeral bone. The engineers, working with a visiting surgeon from the U.S. Navy, cut different-sized lesions into the arm bone and studied how they influenced the shoulder's likelihood of reseparating. The goal was to help devise the most effective—and least invasive—surgical methods to repair these so-called Hill-Sachs lesions.

"If this experiment works, surgeons could make smaller incisions and cause a lot less trauma to the patient," said Jens Stehle, a 31-year-old orthopedic surgeon from Germany and a visiting fellow in Woo's research center. "The shoulder is so much more complicated than the knee. It moves in all directions and is the most dislocated joint in the body. Most of the shoulder's stability is provided by muscles, and there is a very complicated interaction of muscles and the capsule [socket]. This injury is not completely understood, and that's why we're doing these experiments."

On the molecular level, scientists in the Musculoskeletal Research Center are attempting to decode the genetic and cellular mechanisms behind the self-healing properties of the medial collateral ligament. If they can crack that mystery, then they could potentially use that knowledge to treat the anterior cruciate ligament and other ligaments that do not heal on their own.

"We know the MCL healing process works," said Dan Moon, 24, who was getting a master's degree in the center before heading to medical school. "Now we want to work backward and see why it works. This is still at the basic science stage."

An intriguing clue involves the different types of collagen produced in healthy and injured ligaments. Collagen—a tough, fibrous protein that gives tissue its strength—is the main component in ligaments. Connecting bone to bone, ligaments are normally made up largely of a kind of collagen known as "Type I." Injured ligaments contain much more of a collagen known as "Type V," which Woo and his team believe may slow or block the healing process. To speed ligament healing, the scientists are investigating ways to block the production of Type V collagen, perhaps using genetic or cellular therapies. Pitt researchers also have discovered that if they wrap injured MCLs with the sterilized lining of a pig's small intestine and attach the intestinal pig material to the end of the ligament, the MCL heals better and more rapidly as Type V collagen is reduced.

"Twenty years ago research labs in orthopedics focused on joints and mechanics," said Steven D. Abramowitch, an assistant research professor in the Musculoskeletal Research Center. "But to understand what is happening now you have to have a sense of what is going on across the spectrum. You have to understand from the micro to the macro level, from the cells to the whole organ. So you have to collaborate with colleagues in many areas. No one group can do it all."

Woo tries to maintain that balance but stresses to researchers that they must be mindful of the need to move research from bench to bedside.

"We do cellular and molecular research, but we always have function in mind," Woo said as we talked in his office, which overlooks the Monongahela River. "Whatever we do we want to make sure it's ultimately applicable in the clinic. Because we're engineers, we want to make sure it's functional. You can't just do molecular biology without worrying about function. The two have got to meet."

A few miles away, in the Department of Bioengineering's Human Movement and Balance Laboratory, the focus on function and practicality is intense. There, on the main campus of the University of Pittsburgh, investigators such as Rakié Cham, an assistant professor of bioengineering, are investigating basic issues of motility. Chief among them: Why do so many elderly people fall, and what can be done about it?

The problem is large and growing. According to the Centers for Disease Control and Prevention (CDC), in 2001 more than 11,600 Americans over 65 died from injuries sustained in falls. Roughly 1.6 million elderly people went to the emergency room that year after falling, and 388,000 of them were hospitalized. Of that number, about 20 to 30 percent sustained moderate to severe injuries—including hip fractures and head trauma—that often led to extended hospital stays or admission to nursing homes, costing tens of billions of dollars. And the problem, according to the CDC, will only get worse in the coming decades, as the number of people over 65 is expected to more than double, from 35 million in 2000 to 77 million in 2040.

In the Human Movement and Balance Lab, Cham and her colleagues are applying the tools of engineering to study falling in minute detail. On the day I visited, their human guinea pig was 64-year-old Carol Lydon, a slender, athletic woman with five children and ten grandchildren. She had short, pewter-colored hair and blue eyes and was wearing blue spandex shorts and a spandex tank top. Lab workers had affixed seventy-nine marble-sized infrared markers to her body—from her headband to her black leather walking shoes—and hooked her up to a sling harness attached by wires to runners that ran along a steel beam in the ceiling. On the gray linoleum floor were force plates that would record how much force was generated by walking and falling, what researchers call the "kinetics" of gait and falls.

Cham's assistants asked Lydon to walk across the room at a brisk pace, keeping her eyes fixed on the opposite wall. Eight infrared cameras picked up signals from the markers on her body, translating her movements into a three-dimensional computer image. After Lydon walked across the room and returned to her original position, the researchers asked her to turn and face the wall. After the fourth pass, two researchers spread a slippery substance, glycerol, on one of the force plates in Lydon's path. The investigators asked Lydon to turn around and walk across the room again. With her eyes on the opposite wall, she didn't see the glistening floor plate, and as she strode rapidly across it, her foot slipped, her knees buckled, and Lydon fell. The harness caught her. Infrared motion cameras captured the action, while the force plates recorded the kinetics of the fall.

Lydon was one of eighty people involved in the Pitt study, funded by a grant from the National Institute for Occupational Safety and Health. Her fall data and video would be compared with data that measured her strength at different parts of her body and how quickly she was able to muster that strength during exercise. Cham hopes to assemble a detailed picture of the mechanics of falling and what can be done to prevent or lessen the impact of falls, both through exercise and therapy and through improvements in the environment of the elderly.

Cham's group also works with investigators from neighboring Carnegie Mellon University, which uses robots to simulate falls and discover ways to recover from them.

"We're trying to understand why older adults fall more," she said after Lydon had completed her slipping drill. "The things we're looking at are reaction time to the slip, the way they slip, and we try to correlate that with basic health information, such as strength and balance. Once we find out what makes older adults fall more than young people, maybe we can devise some sort of physical training to help prevent falls. Maybe it's mainly a question of reaction time, so we can work on exercises to improve that. Maybe it's mostly a strength issue, and if so, we can work on that."

At the State University of New York, Stony Brook, biomedical engineers are seeking to understand and treat one of the great orthopedic challenges of the twenty-first century: osteoporosis. Marked by a steady decrease in bone mass and density, leading to porous, brittle bones, the disease affects more than 20 million Americans and leads to an estimated $18 billion a year in medical treatment for fractures and related injuries. The U.S. government predicts that by 2025, when many baby boomers are reaching an advanced age, roughly 50 million Americans will have osteoporosis. Many of them will be postmenopausal women, and the consequences of their osteoporosis will lead to tens of billions of dollars more in medical costs if a reliable treatment is not found.

Clinton Rubin, the chairman of the Department of Biomedical Engineering and the director of Stony Brook's Center for Biotechnology, leads a team that has devised a method to treat people with osteoporosis. Realizing that bone is strengthened by muscle tension and movement in a narrow range of electrical energy, Rubin devised a platform that delivers a gentle, high-frequency vibration in that range. Experiments performed by Rubin on both animals and humans have shown that standing on the platform for ten to twenty minutes a day greatly reduces bone loss, which in many postmenopausal women can reach 2 percent per year and which causes hundreds of thousands of bone fractures annually in the United States alone. The National Aeronautics and Space Administration (NASA) was sufficiently impressed with Rubin's experiments that it will test his technology in 2007 on astronauts in the international space station, where weightlessness causes humans to lose bone mass at up to 2 percent per month.

A slender, balding, energetic man in his mid-forties, Rubin has spent more than two decades studying bones and the role that exercise and physical stimulation play in maintaining the skeleton's health. At one point, he considered becoming an architect. When Rubin decided instead to pursue a career in biomedical engineering, he was naturally drawn to the body's superstructure.

"I have always been interested in structure and how structures can withstand loading," said Rubin. "I was intrigued by a smart biomaterial like bone that perceives its environment and adapts to it. And what better designer is there than nature? Bone is a fluid-filled sponge. Bone is not like something in a Georgia O'Keeffe painting, lying out there bleached white in the desert. It is live, viable tissue."

Early in his career, Rubin became fascinated by the close relationship between activity and bone health. A professional tennis player like Venus Williams, for example, has 35 percent greater bone mass in her racket arm than in her other arm. But put people in space, or subject them to debilitating conditions like quadriplegia or cerebral palsy, and their bone mass withers away, leaving them susceptible to fractures. The same is true for the elderly, as the steady decrease in muscle mass and tone leads to a parallel loss in bone mass. Postmenopausal women are especially affected, with the decline of estrogen in the body significantly worsening osteoporosis.

"Muscle is a motor that makes noise, and bone responds to that noise," said Rubin. "As people age, they have less muscle vibration, particularly in the range of 20 to 50 hertz, which is the range that stimulates bone growth. With age this signal falls away, and bone falls away, too."

Rubin's vibrating platform, featured in a 2001 *National Geographic* magazine article on the effect of space flight on humans, has sharply cut the loss of bone density in postmenopausal women and cerebral palsy patients. In a classic exercise in biomedical engineering, Rubin set out to mimic the type of movement that stimulates bone growth and preserves bone density. He wound up inventing a platform a bit larger than a bathroom scale that transmits gentle vibrations through a person's body at thirty cycles per second. His early experiments with the platform involved turkeys, which showed a marked increase in bone density when placed on the device for fifteen to twenty minutes a day for several months.

"What happens as a result of aging, space flight, cerebral palsy, or multiple sclerosis is you lose stimulation in that range, and so we provide a surrogate for it," said Rubin. "We supply something that's missing. That's a simple bioengineering approach to a very complex problem.

"Our group didn't just wake up one day and say, 'Yeah, we could buzz the bone.' We kept asking, 'Could you do this? Could you try that?' We basically whittled away at the problem by looking at the relationship of the cycle, number and frequency of vibrations and the strain on the bone. And we found that bone was more sensitive to high frequency. We found that you don't need to take bone and overpower it with large signals, Whump! Whump! You just need to flutter it. Like a purring cat. That's enough."

To test his vibrating platform, Rubin—in collaboration with Robert Recker, M.D., at the Creighton University Osteoporosis Center in Nebraska—recruited seventy women. They were required to stand on platforms for two ten-minute periods per day. Roughly half stood on actual vibrating platforms, while the other half—the placebo group—stood on platforms that made a humming noise but didn't actually vibrate. Rubin's results, published in 2004, were impressive. Rubin tracked the women for a year, taking a detailed type of X-ray image that showed bone density in their hips and spine. At the end of the year, the members of the placebo group had lost about 3 percent of their bone density, while those in the experimental group had lost less than 1 percent overall, with some even gaining bone mass in their upper spine.

Rubin and a pediatrician from England, Zulf Mughal, performed a similar experiment with twenty children, ages 9 to 16, with cerebral palsy. The study showed that after six months the group that had been on the vibrating platform actually had a 6 percent gain in bone density, while the placebo group experienced a 10 percent loss in bone mass. People with cerebral palsy, who often are restricted to wheelchairs because of impaired motor function and lack of muscle control, frequently experience "spontaneous" fractures, with little cause, because of osteoporosis.

Rubin's device has not yet been approved by the FDA, and clinical trials are continuing. But his results have attracted the attention of NASA, which during a 2007 stay on the International Space Station will use the vibrating platform to study its impact on astronauts.

Drugs have had some success in stemming osteoporosis. One type blocks the production of osteoclasts, cells that reabsorb bone and can cause osteoporosis if they become more active than bone-producing cells, known as osteoblasts. A second type of drug stimulates the production of osteoblasts to slow osteoporosis. But Rubin said the long-term effects of these drugs are unknown, making a simpler approach, like the vibrating platform, more appealing.

In Rubin's department, as in all of biomedical engineering, the search for treatments is advancing to the level of genes and molecules. One associate professor, Stefan Judex, is conducting an exhaustive study of mice to try to find the region on the mouse genome—which is extremely similar to the human genome—that sends out the signals setting osteoporosis in motion.

Judex has no doubt that genes play a part in osteoporosis. Among astronauts in space, for example, bone loss is highly variable, even though the astronauts are subjected to the same diet and exercise regime. Such variability is also observed in postmenopausal women. In order to explore the role of genetics in osteoporosis, Judex is exposing more than 500 genetically heterogeneous mice to conditions of simulated weightlessness. He does so by suspending the mice in cages from their tail, allowing their front legs to firmly touch the ground, while the hind legs barely brush the bottom of the cage. Using a powerful micro-CT scanner, Judex then studies changes in the femur bones over a three-week period. A major reason Judex can perform this study is because of engineering-driven improvements in imaging in recent years. Micro-CT scanners can now produce a three-dimensional bone scan of a mouse that is ten times more powerful than a CT scan used in human clinics and can deliver and reconstruct those images in real time. The images have a resolution of about 10 microns, fine enough to discern very small anatomical features, even in mouse bones.

After testing more than 300 mice with different genetic makeups, Judex discovered that some of the animals lost only 15 to 20 percent of their bone density, while many animals lost 60 percent, with some even experiencing declines of 88 percent. His intention is to separate out the mice highly prone to osteoporosis, and those that are highly resistant, and study differences in their genetic makeup by genotyping their chromosomes.

"We look at large chunks of DNA spanning hundreds or thousands of genes," said Judex, a tall, fit German in his mid-thirties who often jogs to and from his office. "We want to see the genetic differences among these strains. At this point, we can't bring it down to one gene, but we can say that the reason this mouse responds differently from that mouse is because of polymorphisms [differences] in this region of the genome."

Since mice and humans share more than 95 percent of their genes, the mouse research will no doubt be valuable in attacking osteoporosis in humans. And Judex eventually wants to perform genetic studies on humans, including astronauts.

"Bone loss among individuals varies tremendously, and obviously genetics plays a part," said Judex. "The big picture is we'll try to identify those people most prone to bone loss. We will start with astronauts, but our approach can also be applied to postmenopausal women. The ultimate goal is to find some sort of intervention, perhaps tailored to an individual's genetic makeup, that will slow or stop that loss."

Said Rubin, "Stefan could well find the area of the genome that makes you osteoporotic."

If that occurs, the goal in the long run would be to come up with a genetic or drug therapy that would safely block the genes that play a role in osteoporosis.

One of Judex's colleagues in the Department of Biomedical Engineering, Associate Professor Michael Hadjiargyrou, is also deep into genetic studies, although with a different aim: identifying the genes involved in bone fracture repair and using that knowledge to speed the healing process, fix fractures resistant to normal treatment, and replace bone lost to cancer. To date, Hadjiargyrou and the researchers in his lab have done the equivalent of assembling the pieces of a giant jigsaw puzzle of genetic information. By creating fractures in the femurs of rats and then looking at the genes that are turned on to help repair the fracture over the course of three weeks, Hadjiargyrou has identified thousands of genes possibly involved in healing broken bone. He has a good idea of which genes are especially active and has even identified one factor—activated by a low concentration of oxygen—that seems to play a vital role in creating the blood vessels that help repair bone.

Still, Hadjiargyrou and his research group are a long way from assembling a complete picture and understanding the hundreds of genes involved in the repair process and their interactions. But Hadjiargyrou is optimistic that he and other researchers will one day piece together a portrait of the bone repair process, opening the way for numerous therapies. One he is currently investigating is placing DNA that speeds bone repair into biodegradable scaffolds and then implanting those scaffolds at fracture sites. Such a treatment could significantly aid the healing process and may well fix the 10 percent of fractures that never properly fuse.

"You take an adult who has to wear a cast now for six weeks, and we throw in one of these scaffolds that heals the fracture two to three times faster, then you've got someone going back to work in two weeks, not six weeks," said Hadjiargyrou.

Hadjiargyrou's work, combining a biomedical device—a degradable scaffold—with genetic therapy, offers a glimpse of where Rubin sees the field heading in the future.

"It would be a snub to the tradition of biomedical engineering to abandon its roots in devices," said Rubin. "Biomedical engineering should be all of these things. It will be a leader in functional devices and also in genomics, where there are big computational problems that are well suited to bioengineers. But this can't be done by sacrificing our traditional role in diagnostics and intervention. We'll grow into new fields without abandoning the old ones."

Chapter 11

The Pictures

Like many women with breast cancer, Teresa Powell soon came to understand that fighting the disease was a running battle. The 48-year-old mother of two from northern California was first diagnosed with a marble-sized tumor in her right breast in 1997. Surgeons removed the cancer, in a procedure known as a lumpectomy. Three years later, the cancer returned and was surgically removed again. Powell also received a round of radiation treatments. But by the summer of 2004, the cancer was back, and this time doctors were concerned that it might have spread beyond her right breast.

Seeking to determine whether her cancer had metastasized, Powell's physicians recommended that she visit the Cancer Center at the University of California, Davis. Located in Sacramento, the UC Davis center recently had installed an imaging system, known as a PET-CT scanner, that would scrutinize her entire body and, in about half an hour, tell doctors whether and where cancerous growths had taken up residence.

On a cold, overcast morning several weeks before Christmas in 2004, Powell arrived at the UC Davis Medical Center for her scan. There, in the Department of Radiology, a nurse injected her with a radioactive tracer called fluorodeoxyglucose, known as FDG. The FDG, one of a growing number of compounds called molecular tracers, or probes, would course through Powell's body for a few hours before disappearing. The molecular structure of FDG makes it a unique tool in the arsenal of weapons used to detect cancer. FDG enters all the cells in the body but accumulates in those burning a lot of glucose, lighting them up with minute quantities of radioactivity. When passed through a PET (positron emission tomography) scanner, Powell's brain would show up as a dark blotch on the computer because its active metabolism burns glucose. So would her heart, kidneys, and bladder. And so would clusters of cancer cells, which consume large amounts of glucose as they divide and multiply out of control.

"FDG is amazing," explained Simon Cherry, a professor of biomedical engineering at UC Davis and a leading PET researcher. "The cancer soaks up the radioactive glucose, and out of the fog emerge hot spots showing the location of the cancer."

At 11:20 a.m., Powell was rolled in a wheelchair from the Radiology Department to a gleaming white trailer parked in a lot behind the medical center. Inside was a large, light gray PET-CT scanner made by GE Healthcare. A technologist placed Powell on her back on a narrow bed and prepared to run her through the first phase of the scan. The CT scan—also known as a CAT (computerized axial tomography) scan—worked by beaming X-rays through Powell's body. However, instead of taking a single X-ray image, like a conventional X-ray machine in the ER or a dental practice, the CT scanner projected radiation through Powell's body from a full 360-degree range of angles. On the opposite side of the X-ray emitter were a series of detectors that would read the beams after they passed through the tissues in Powell's body. But what really distinguished a CT scan from a regular X-ray was massive computing power. All the pictures taken by the CT machine were fed into a computer, which assembled them, slice by slice, into a three-dimensional view of Powell's insides.

"Okay, here we go," Howard Carpenter, a fifth-year resident in radiological and nuclear medicine, said to Powell. "Breathe in. . . . Breathe out. . . . Now stop breathing."

Fourteen seconds later, the CT scanner had taken its pictures—about ten times faster than CT machines a decade before. The processed images would give Carpenter and Powell's personal physician a detailed anatomical view of the woman's body, including any sizable tumors. But as good as the CT scan was, it showed only anatomy, not the actual physiological functions of tissues and organs. And to get a sense of where cancer is lurking in the body, nothing could top the PET scan, which would pinpoint the glucose-burning cancer hot spots inside Powell.

For her PET scan, Powell lay in the same open-ended machine used for the CT image. While CT scans and X-rays beam radiation at a person from the outside in, a PET scan works in opposite fashion, from the inside out, with rapidly decaying radioactive atoms inside the patient emitting signals picked up by a ring of detectors. As Powell's scan began, the decaying radioactivity trapped inside her tumor cells emitted atomic particles called positrons, which collided with electrons, annihilating both. Each of those destructive collisions produced two photons that shot out in diametrically opposite directions. Millions of these photons were spewed out every second from the radioactive FDG molecules inside Powell, striking the PET machine's detectors. Then, crunching about 100 million pieces of data, the PET scanner's computers produced an image showing spots in Powell's body metabolizing large amounts of glucose.

The drawback of the PET scan was that, while it vividly highlighted tumors, there was no way of telling their precise location. That's where the CT scan, which provides a precise map of Powell's anatomy, came in. By superimposing the PET and CT images on each other, the GE machine's computer was able to produce a crisp picture showing the exact size and location of the cancer.

For Powell, the results of the scan were mixed. Her cancer had spread from a tumor on the outer side of her right breast into a series of lymph nodes in the same breast. The combined PET-CT image showed normal tissues in various shades of red, yellow, orange, and gray, while the cancerous lymph nodes were a line of bright circles stretching across half her chest. (Tissue biopsies later confirmed that the cancer had spread to seven lymph nodes in her breast and armpit.) But the PET scan also showed that the cancer had not metastasized to other parts of her body. A month after her scan, Powell's doctors performed a mastectomy and removed her right breast. They also removed a series of lymph nodes under her arm, and shortly afterward she began a round of chemotherapy to prevent the further spread or return of the disease.

Powell, who cleans houses near the town of Auburn, California, about 35 miles northeast of Sacramento, said she was grateful that a technology like PET made it possible to detect the spread of cancer. In her case, PET provided a measure of relief.

"They said this would definitely show if it had spread," said Powell. "It's the newest thing. Obviously I didn't understand it all. . . . But I feel healthy. And I hope they find a cure for me and everyone else."

The technique used to monitor Teresa Powell's cancer provides a glimpse into where medical imaging has been and where it's heading. Of all biomedical engineering's achievements, few have matched the rapid advances of imaging, which have enabled doctors to peer inside the body without lifting a scalpel. For more than half a century after the discovery of the X-ray by German physicist Wilhelm Roentgen in 1895, that technology was the only method doctors possessed to image a patient. Although great for spotting a broken bone, a large tumor, or an area of tuberculosis on the lung, the X-ray had severe limitations, most notably its inability to accurately depict soft tissues or show how organs like the brain were actually functioning.

In the decades after World War II, however, a host of new imaging technologies came on the scene, and soon the state of the art—the X-ray—was being surpassed by numerous new machines. Ultrasound, an outgrowth of sonar technology used to detect submarines, gave doctors the ability to see a fetus developing inside the womb or a heart defect in a patient. CT scans, though crude and slow in the beginning, gave physicians a detailed look at internal organs such as the kidney and liver. And magnetic resonance imaging—known as MRI—relied on the different magnetic properties of various atoms in the body to create a whole new way of imaging, one that was superb at distinguishing function and abnormalities in the body's soft tissues, such as the brain.

In the past decade or two, as dizzying leaps have been made in computing power, semiconductor technology, and microelectronics, these new imaging techniques have all become faster and more accurate. They are an essential part of making many medical diagnoses, taking their place alongside other indispensable imaging techniques such as angiography, which involves injecting radioactive dye into patients to assess the state of their arteries and heart. In 2004, Americans underwent 58 million CT scans, 23 million MRIs, and 120 million X-rays. Today, the cost of running tens of millions of patients through these advanced scanners exceeds $100 billion. Insurance companies and HMOs, alarmed by soaring imaging costs, are fighting to reduce the number of inappropriate or unnecessary scans.

But despite the enormous expense, no one would dispute the value of imaging, a field that has leapt forward thanks to the research efforts of biomedical engineers, electrical engineers, physicists, and doctors. As Martin Yarmush, chairman of the Department of Biomedical Engineering at Rutgers University, said, "If you have to say what biomedical engineering has done above all, it's imaging. That's number one. It has revolutionized medicine. These tools have allowed us to look inside the body without cutting it open."

Bob Armstrong, general manager of Global Functional and CT Engineering for GE Healthcare, America's biggest maker of medical imaging machines, said that the costs of imaging must be weighed against what came before.

"What diagnostic imaging brings is the opportunity for the medical community to have noninvasive, diagnostic certainty," said Armstrong. "If you ask me about costs, let's go back to before any of this was around. Imagine if we brought exploratory surgery back, with all the operating time and long hospital stays."

As revolutionary as recent imaging advances have been, the field is now on the threshold of developments that may one day make conventional CT and MRI scans look primitive. This new frontier is known as molecular imaging, and its goal is to be able to target, visualize, and then treat disease on the cellular and molecular level, opening up what physicians and biomedical engineers say will be individually tailored treatments for diseases like cancer. Teresa Powell's PET scan, which relied on the ability of the radioactive tracer FDG to be taken up into cells just like natural glucose, is the latest and most common molecular imaging technique to achieve widespread clinical use. But researchers around the globe are rapidly developing new probes, tracers, and other ways of imaging cells.

The director of the UC Davis Cancer Center, Ralph deVere White, said his institution, like hundreds around the country and the world, is venturing into uncharted territory. But he is certain of the outcome. The progress in molecular imaging and molecular medicine will eventually make today's diagnosis and treatment of cancer look woefully inadequate. DeVere White and others believe that cancer—now the leading killer of Americans, taking nearly 500,000 lives in 2004—will one day become more of a chronic affliction, as cardiovascular disease is today.

"Today's care will be distant history," said deVere White. "It will look like the big room of computers that existed in the 1960s. Yes, those computers worked and people did their best. But compared to a laptop computer, which can do the same work, that roomful of computers is ancient history."

To date, most advances in imaging have been focused on rapidly improving the speed and resolution of scans, enabling doctors to see ever smaller aspects of physiology with ever faster scans. But seeing the structure of the body in detail can advance medicine only so far, said Armstrong. What's needed now, and where imaging is headed, is characterizing the body's functions on a molecular level, opening the way to treat diseases, such as cancer, at their weakest points.

"If you think about what the future holds, all these imaging technologies have been based around structure and applying different physics and methods to look at structure," said Armstrong. "But one must truly ask how much structure is enough? Does it matter? You can now see things on images that are so small you can't even biopsy them. Our ability to see things has outstripped our ability to characterize what we're seeing. Engineering and technology always drive us to faster scans and better resolution, but we have to ask the question, do we care? We have to go beyond structure. We have to go to function, and PET and nuclear medicine is all about function. The future is about how we move beyond structure to function. We're going to reinvent the entire industry around this."

The slowly unfolding shift from imaging bones, tissue, and organs to imaging on the molecular and cellular level is representative of a sweeping change taking place in all of biomedical engineering. Increasingly, the thrust of research in the field is going from big to small, from devices that assist or replace diseased organs, joints, and other body parts to therapies that manipulate the very basis of life—molecules, genes, and proteins. Many biomedical engineers, particularly younger ones swept up in the genetic and biological revolutions, want to understand what makes the body tick at its most fundamental level. It was inevitable, then, that imaging would move down the same path.

The University of California, Davis, is home to a recently created Department of Biomedical Engineering that hopes to make its name in the new world of molecular imaging. Established in 2001 and led initially by chairwoman Katherine W. Ferrara, the department hopes to make its name in the new world of molecular imaging, and many of its dozen faculty members are conducting research into this new field, working in a new genomic and biomedical sciences building dedicated in 2004. The basement contains some of the most up-to-date experimental imaging equipment in the country, including a cyclotron to make radioactive isotopes, several microPET machines to image mice, and an array of CT, MRI, and ultrasound scanners, as well as optical imaging equipment that may be able to tell whether a cell is cancerous just by scanning it with a laser.

The guiding theory behind molecular imaging is a simple one. Diseased cells, such as cancer cells, have a definite signature and produce certain kinds of enzymes, growth factors, and other substances. Tumors, for example, need new blood vessels to keep expanding, and those blood vessels generate a particular growth factor as they form. The aim of molecular imaging and molecular medicine is to introduce substances into a patient's body designed to lock on to those enzymes and growth factors and through them to kill or block the growth of diseased cells. Isotopes and tracers can affix themselves to the cells and identify them to an imaging machine, after which drugs or genetic therapies can be used to find and destroy certain cell types.

With cancer, for example, different tumors send out different signals, meaning an array of probes or tracers will have to be devised to track down the many varieties of cancer. In addition, an individual's genetic makeup makes him or her more likely to be stricken with a certain disease and to react differently to therapies. The overarching goal is to determine, through genetic screening, which therapies are best suited to different individuals, a strategy that is already being applied to women with certain breast cancers.

Molecular imaging will play a central role in this new phase of diagnosing and treating diseases. That became evident to me on my first day at UC Davis, when Ferrara took me to a meeting at the university's cancer center in Sacramento, 15 miles east of the Davis campus. Arrayed around a long, oval table in a conference room were about twenty doctors, biomedical engineers, and physicists. They were part of UC Davis's Cancer Therapeutics Working Group, which pulls in experts from many disciplines to conduct trials in molecular imaging and targeted molecular drug therapy. The group discussed some of the better-known drugs, such as Iressa and Gleevec, which lock on to certain molecules to kill cancer cells. They also discussed results of trials with some newer agents, such as a compound called AZD2171, made by AstraZeneca. This compound inhibits a growth factor, known as VEGF, that helps blood vessels spread in tumors.

"These are the hot drugs," Dr. David Gandara, the cancer center's associate director of clinical research, told the gathering. "There will be a move away from chemotherapy, radiation, and even surgery, toward these targeted molecular agents. You can look for markers on tumors, image them, and then modify or continue therapy."

Ramsey D. Badawi, an assistant professor in the Department of Radiology who is working closely with Ferrara's department on PET research, added, "The next ten years will be about functional molecular imaging."

Badawi then flashed several images on a screen to demonstrate the power of molecular imaging. The images were from a patient who had received molecular therapy for a rare type of intestinal cancer. Before treatment, the patient had a PET scan that showed huge amounts of disease throughout the body. The day after the therapy started, the patient had another PET scan, which showed a massive reduction in the amount of glucose the diseased tissues were using, indicating that the therapy was already working. The case demonstrated molecular imaging's superior potential, as compared with CT or MR imaging, to measure the body's response to therapy.

"These results could never be found so early with a CT scan," Badawi said later. "Anatomic changes simply don't happen that fast."

This is only the beginning, Badawi said, of what molecular imaging can accomplish.

Already, biomedical engineers and other researchers are developing molecular probes that could one day prove valuable in imaging the brains of people in the early stages of diseases such as Parkinson's and Alzheimer's. Investigators have devised a radioactive compound, called fluorodopa, that attaches to cells producing dopamine, a neurotransmitter essential in basic movement. This could identify patients with a lack of dopamine, which causes Parkinson's symptoms such as tremors and difficulty moving. Early diagnosis of dopamine deficiencies could open the door to more effective treatment with drugs or other therapies.

The same is true of Alzheimer's disease. At the University of California, Los Angeles, researchers have produced a radioactive compound, known as FDDNP, that locks on to the amyloid plaques that gum up the brains of Alzheimer's patients. By using PET scans and radiopharmaceuticals to screen patients showing signs of memory lapses, physicians could determine which people are merely experiencing normal, age-related memory loss and which seem to be on the road to developing full-blown Alzheimer's. Although no highly effective Alzheimer's drug treatments have yet been devised, various probes could one day be used to deliver drug payloads that would seek and destroy the tangled, amyloid proteins in the brains of people with Alzheimer's. FDG also can be effective in helping diagnose

Alzheimer's, since people with the disease have reduced brain function, leading to lower glucose metabolism.

Radioactive tracers are vital to the new molecular medicine, and though a probe like FDG was first developed several decades ago, physicians and researchers are just beginning to grasp its import. As Badawi, who has been instrumental in setting up UC Davis's PET imaging center, said, "A tracer is like smoke in a wind tunnel. It's something you can see but does not interfere with what you're measuring. It musn't perturb the process but must genuinely track it. This has been going on for thirty years. But now people have discovered that 'Wow! This is where it's really at.'"

Other sophisticated probes and tracers are being developed on the genetic level, as researchers design so-called reporter genes that will fluoresce or trap radioactive tracers and identify themselves inside cells. The technique of inserting reporter genes in cells is important not only for research but also for gene therapy, if and when it proves safe to begin manipulating genes in human beings to treat disease.

"Basically the horizon is limitless," said Dr. Gary Caputo, a professor of clinical radiology at UC Davis. "Molecular imaging will be a fascinating area. It will be a toolbox you can just reach into."

CHAPTER 12

Seeing the Unseen

German physicist Wilhelm Roentgen was the first to discover the paradox of medical imaging: that invisible energy could make the unseen visible. His discovery came quite by accident. On November 8, 1895, Roentgen was studying electrons generated in a vacuum cathode ray tube. In a nearby room was a sheet of paper covered with barium platinocyanide, a substance used for coating some types of photographic plates. Glancing at the paper, he noticed that it had a fluorescent glow and realized that an invisible ray emitted by the cathode tube had imprinted an image on the paper. He had no idea what the rays were, hence the name X-ray. But he soon understood that he had stumbled upon a major scientific discovery, one that enabled doctors to see inside the body with a mysterious energy that passed through flesh but was blocked by bone. In short order, he aimed the cathode ray tube at a sheet of coated paper and instructed his wife to place her hand in front of the paper. In doing so, Roentgen created the first medical radiograph, which showed the dark bones and ring on her hand.

Within a year of Roentgen's discovery, both General Electric (GE) and Siemens began manufacturing X-ray machines for hospitals. The impact on medicine cannot be overstated, as doctors now had the ability to see, from the outside, a broken bone, a bullet, or a tumor on a lung. In the first few decades of the twentieth century, engineers at GE and various research institutions greatly improved the quality of X-rays, lowering the doses of harmful radiation while enhancing the machine's ability to image some soft tissue. Other researchers discovered that they could image patients' digestive tract by having them ingest mildly radioactive compounds, such as bismuth or barium, and then taking X-rays of their torso. Another major breakthrough came in the 1920s when Portuguese researchers discovered that by injecting radioactive substances into patients' veins, doctors could obtain pictures of the cardiovascular system. This was the birth of angiography, which did not come into widespread clinical use for several more decades.

The next major medical imaging advance came in the 1940s, this time when engineers used another invisible form of energy—sound waves—to look inside the human body. Sonar, which emitted sound waves to detect submarines, was invented at the end of World War I, and in 1941 British engineer Donald Sproule devised the precursor of the modern medical ultrasound machine, which contained a transducer that sent out a pulse of sound and a receiver that recorded the echoes. The sound waves bounced off tissues of varying densities in different ways, enabling doctors in those early years to get a fuzzy image of a person's insides. Human ultrasound began to move into clinical practice in the 1950s and 1960s, and the clarity of its images steadily improved with the miniaturization of electronics. Today, as many as 200 transducers send out sound pulses, compared with a dozen two decades ago. These new machines provide far sharper images, whether of a developing fetus or of a beating heart.

In the early 1950s, Hal Anger, a physicist at the University of California, Berkeley, developed the gamma camera, which took pictures of the distribution of radioactivity within the body. Anger's invention was the beginning of nuclear medicine, which employs mildly radioactive contrast agents to see inside the body. Now used in every major hospital, nuclear medicine paved the way for such common procedures as cardiac catheterization to measure arterial blockages. The gamma camera also was the first molecular imaging technique and an early precursor to PET scanners.

The CT scanner was invented in the early 1970s by a number of researchers working independently in the United States and England. One of the leading inventors was Godfrey Hounsfield, an English electrical engineer who, along with Allan Cormack, was awarded the 1979 Nobel Prize in Medicine for inventing the CT scan. The key element of their invention was the concept of passing a person through a circular scanner that would shoot X-ray pictures from many perspectives.

"The breakthrough was the realization that by scanning objects at many angles, it was possible to extract 100 percent of information," Hounsfield said in a 1973 interview with the *New York Times.*

The myriad X-rays, combined by the computer into a two-dimensional image, enabled doctors to see tissue in great detail. Previously, for example, X-rays would show only a person's skull, not whether there was a tumor or bleeding in the brain. The CT scan could show it all, for its rays were not blocked by bone, as were the sound waves of ultrasound.

In its award presentation, the Nobel Committee said that "ordinary X-ray examinations of the head had shown the skull bones, but the brain had remained a gray, undifferentiated fog. Now suddenly the fog had cleared."

In the early 1970s, other scientists and engineers also developed a second powerful imaging technique that has revolutionized medical diagnostics: magnetic resonance imaging. As early as the 1930s, scientists had discovered that when subjected to strong magnetic fields, atoms snap into magnetic alignment and give off radio signals. When the magnetic pulse is turned off, the atoms relax, also emitting radio signals in the process. In the late 1960s and early 1970s, several scientists, working independently, figured out that this magnetic property of atoms could be a sound basis for imaging, as different elements of the body—blood, soft tissue, ligaments, spinal fluid, tumors—all gave off different radio signals when magnetic fields were turned on and off. (The most common atom imaged by MRI is hydrogen, part of the water that constitutes most of the human body.) The pioneers in MRI were Paul C. Lauterbur of the State University of New York at Stony Brook; Sir Peter Mansfield of the University of Nottingham in England; and Raymond Damadian of the State University of New York Downstate Medical Center. In 2003, Lauterbur and Mansfield were awarded the Nobel Prize in Medicine for inventing MRI. Damadian was overlooked, prompting him and his supporters to launch a nationwide campaign—including full-page ads in the *New York Times*—to persuade the Nobel Committee to also award the prize to Damadian.

Both CT and MRI scans came into wide clinical use in the early 1980s. The MRI scan has had incalculable value, enabling orthopedists to image torn ligaments and tendons, back specialists to see ruptured disks and the spinal column pressing on nerves, and oncologists to get a clear picture of tumors. MRIs have proven extremely valuable in neurology, especially with the advent of what is known as functional magnetic resonance imaging (fMRI). This involves imaging the metabolism and blood flow of the brain, enabling neurologists and psychiatrists to see the physical anomalies associated with such diseases as multiple sclerosis, Alzheimer's, and schizophrenia.

Engineers and researchers have continued to improve MRI and CT scans, steadily increasing their speed thanks primarily to great leaps in computing power. Moore's law, named for Intel co-founder Gordon Moore, states that the number of transistors on an integrated circuit—and hence the speed of computer processors—doubles every year. That axiom has held true for imaging, where scanning speeds have been increasing at about the same rate.

In addition, the miniaturization of electronics has enabled engineers to place far more transducers and detection cells on imaging machines, greatly boosting resolution. Bob Armstrong of GE Healthcare cited just one example of the field's relentless progress. In 1984, when Armstrong first began working for GE, a CT scan of the human body would take thirty minutes, would image slices of the body that were eight-tenths of an inch thick, and would generate about thirty images for doctors to examine. Today, a full-body CT scan takes thirty seconds, shoots images of the body as thin as a credit card, and generates about 2,000 images, which computers assemble into a highly detailed view of the body from top to bottom. In 1984, a busy CT clinic would scan ten people per day. Now, that same clinic can comfortably image 60 to 80 people in a day.

"Speed and resolution," said Armstrong, "have driven diagnostic imaging."

Currently, biomedical and computer engineers are tackling one of the major drawbacks of CT, which is its difficulty taking sharp pictures of the beating heart. The motion of the heart, and its varying rate, create blurry CT images, an obstacle investigators are attempting to overcome by devising new computer algorithms.

Another major drawback of CT is that it uses ionizing radiation, and Armstrong said GE and other imaging companies are laboring to create CT scanners that retain today's high-quality images while significantly reducing the radiation dose beamed through the patient.

"Look, I love CT—every human being ought to love CT because it got rid of exploratory surgery," said Armstrong. "But CT's number one virtue is also its number one liability, and that is that it uses X-rays."

Like CT scans, ultrasound scanning has undergone a similar revolution in image quality. Fifteen years ago, when an obstetrician performed an in utero ultrasound scan of the oldest of Armstrong's three children, the black-and-white images were blurry, almost "like a Rorschach test," he said. Today, however, parents seeing an ultrasound of their baby in the womb are treated to three-dimensional color images of remarkable clarity, leaving no doubt, as there once was, whether it is a boy or a girl.

"They're beautiful now, almost like the photographs of fetuses you used to see in *Life* magazine," said Armstrong. "They're incredible."

In MRI technology, advances in computer speeds have made it possible to generate real-time images. In addition, engineers are employing ever more powerful magnets in MRI machines, with a force tens of thousands of times stronger than the earth's magnetic field, to create finer resolution.

Some biomedical engineers and physicians, such as James Brookeman of the University of Virginia, are using a new technique for lung imaging that has drastically improved pulmonary MRI scans. This involves inhaling gases, such as xenon or helium, that have been hyperpolarized, which makes them especially sensitive to magnetism and thus an excellent contrast agent. The quality of the images is superb, as I learned when I met Brookeman, who showed me a series of MR images on his computer. In a healthy person, the many alveoli in the lungs, where the blood absorbs oxygen from the air, were clearly visible, forming a light gray image of the entire lung. But the images of smokers with emphysema were riddled with countless dark regions, representing dead zones where the hyperpolarized gas could not penetrate.

Looking back, the great advances in CT and MR imaging in the 1970s and 1980s represented a golden age in the field, one that fundamentally altered the practice of medicine worldwide. As Dr. William Hendee, an imaging expert who is dean of research in the Department of Radiology at the Medical College of Wisconsin, put it, "It was a technological revolution. It's like before the development of the interstate highway system and after the development of the interstate."

Today, molecular imaging is poised to make as big a leap.

The new Genome and Biomedical Sciences building at the University of California, Davis, sits on the outskirts of the laid-back town of Davis, adjacent to the university's medical school. When I visited UC Davis—one of ten schools in the University of California system—in December 2004, the six-story, 225,000-square-foot building was still surrounded by swaths of unlandscaped dirt and gravel. But the students and faculty had moved into offices on the second and third floors and were relishing the expansiveness of their new quarters.

One afternoon, I spent time in Simon Cherry's lab observing the research of two graduate students working on technology to create a combined PET-MRI scanner. The task was daunting, if for no other reason than the PET equipment could contain no metal because of the powerful magnets used in the MRI. But the students, Jennifer Stickel and Ciprian Catana, were experimenting with a possible solution. Building on the work of other scientists, they were creating what they hoped would be a highly sensitive cluster of inorganic crystal detectors designed to pick up the photons as they shot out, at a rate of millions per second, from the radionuclides inside a patient's body. Older detectors, a little less than an inch on each side, had 64 crystals fused together. But Stickel and Catana were experimenting with a detector containing 1,200 crystals in the same space. Because it possessed so many crystals, the detector could more accurately pinpoint the location of positrons emitted from the person's body. The device was a marvel of miniaturization, with each crystal converting the energy of the photons into light, and then electricity, using photo multiplier tubes.

I watched as the two students placed the detector in a metal box the size of a small refrigerator. Inside the box was a small sample of sodium-22, a radionuclide that would, as it decayed, beam photons at the new detector. The experiment began, and a red-orange blur appeared on a computer screen. This was the detector picking up the photons, but rather than seeing hundreds of distinct dots, each representing a signal from an individual crystal, Stickel and Catana wound up with little more than a colorful smudge. They soon figured out that the optical gel they had put on their detector to enhance performance had had the opposite effect. So they wiped the detector clean and, in a few minutes, received an image in which some of the individual crystals showed up as distinct points of color. Still, the 1,200 crystals were so close together that the scientists were a long way from getting a sharp signal from each one—their ultimate aim.

For Stickel, this was precisely the kind of challenge—combining medicine, math, computer science, and electrical engineering—that drew her to biomedical engineering in the first place.

"In high school, I didn't want to just do biology," said Stickel, who has an undergraduate degree in biomedical engineering from Boston University. "There wasn't enough math, and there was too much rote memorization. I found it fascinating that people were applying engineering to biology. My mom was a nurse, and I was just interested in what goes on in the body and how you measure it. Biomedical engineering just seemed a lot more quantitative."

Stickel is especially intrigued by molecular imaging. One area that interests her is the diagnosis and treatment of breast cancer. She noted that breast cancer cells rely on the hormone estrogen to survive and grow. Indeed, scientists have discovered that breast cancer cells have nearly 400 times the number of estrogen receptors on their surface that normal cells have. The challenge, said Stickel, is to find a molecular tracer that will bind to these estrogen receptors so that the breast cancer cells can be imaged and ultimately targeted for destruction.

"It won't just be a doctor saying. 'Go get a CT or an MRI,'" said Stickel. "It will be a doctor saying, 'You have breast cancer, this is what kind you have, and this is what will be the best treatment for you.' Imaging and medicine will be a lot more tailored to the individual. There will be a real merging of molecular biology and noninvasive imaging techniques. I see medicine becoming more and more preventative."

In a nearby lab, Assistant Professor Angelique Louie is working on another promising area of molecular imaging, which would use MRI technology to target the plaques that build up in arteries. Her goal is to find an agent that would attach itself to macrophages, the large white blood cells that play an important role in plaque formation. To do this, Louie needs to find a molecule or compound that would not only lock on to the hundreds of thousands of receptors found in each macrophage but would also contain tracers that would highlight the macrophages—and hence the plaques—on an MRI scan. Such a binding mechanism also could theoretically be used to deliver drugs or other therapies to bust up the plaques.

Much of UC Davis's research into molecular imaging takes place in the basement, where the Biomedical Engineering Department has set up extensive labs for imaging mice, some 20,000 of which can be housed in the basement's vivarium. Cherry has invented a machine known as the microPET II, designed to run molecular imaging tests on mice. It is a vast improvement over previous, small-animal PET scanners, with an eightfold increase in resolution and the ability to image tumors as small as 1 square millimeter. Having machines to perform precise PET scans on mice is a boon to research, since nearly all the investigations done into cancer and other diseases use mice, which share about 95 percent of their genes with humans.

"Imaging provides a way to track the development of the disease and to evaluate new therapeutic approaches in living animals and follow time courses with individual animals," said Cherry.

Adjacent to the microPET lab is the cyclotron, the domain of Julie Sutcliffe-Goulden, assistant professor of biomedical engineering. A native of England, Sutcliffe-Goulden was hired to oversee work with the cyclotron, a $2 million machine that manufactures radioactive isotopes used in molecular imaging. Among the isotopes she will be creating are fluorine-18, carbon-11, oxygen-15, and nitrogen-13. Each isotope has a different rate of decay, which is known as its half-life. So far FDG—labeled with fluorine-18, which has a half-life of 110 minutes—has proved to be the best radioactive tracer yet used in molecular medicine. But Sutcliffe-Goulden, in collaboration with researchers at the UC Davis Cancer Center, is working to come up with new radioactive tracers to expand the reach of molecular imaging.

"For me, I have to see it leave the lab bench and have value to the patients," said Sutcliffe-Goulden.

Helping her do that is Kit S. Lam, chief of UC Davis's Division of Hematology and Oncology. Lam undertakes research in a field known as "combinatorial chemistry," which uses powerful computers to test permutations of thousands of molecules to see which might be employed to image and attack cancer on a molecular or genetic level. Lam's work is similar to that done by pharmaceutical companies when they use massive computing power to combine tens of thousands of different molecules and compounds to come up with new drugs. "The mechanism of how molecular imaging works is very similar to the way a drug works," said Lam.

One recent example of targeted molecular cancer therapy is Zevalin, made by Biogen Idec. Zevalin, used to treat non-Hodgkin's lymphoma, employs radioactive antibodies to seek out receptors on lymphoma cells and then releases radiation to kill the cells. An often used analogy in such therapies is that the antibodies are like keys that open the locks, or receptors, to targeted cells.

"Now we better understand cancer and how it forms," said Lam. "Twenty years ago it was a big black box. Now it's not. The challenge is finding the molecules that target those pathways. The Holy Grail is to find a molecule that binds to a specific DNA sequence."

Although molecular imaging may represent the future of the field, investigators in UC Davis's Department of Biomedical Engineering also are working to push traditional imaging technologies in new directions. One of the most prominent researchers is Professor John M. Boone, who has spent five years developing a breast CT scanner that promises to be significantly more sensitive than X-ray mammography.

Mammography, the current gold standard for breast cancer screening, detects tumors that average 11 millimeters in diameter, or about half an inch. A mammogram usually consists of two X-ray images, providing a two-dimensional picture. With mammography, a woman's fatty tissue and glandular structures sometimes block tumors from sight. Traditional CT scans of the upper torso provide a three-dimensional view of the breast, but it is of low resolution. Another drawback of traditional, full-body CT scans is that they subject breast cancer patients to more radiation than is necessary, since the X-rays have to pass through the torso, not just the breast.

Boone, who has a Ph.D. in medical physics, believed there had to be a way to devise a CT scan just for the breast, and in 1997 he set to work. With grants from the National Institutes of Health (NIH) and the state of California, his lab has invented and built a new CT scanner that is expected to enable physicians to detect smaller tumors at an earlier stage. Such an advance could save thousands of lives a year, as breast cancer, like nearly all cancers, is far easier to treat in its beginning stages.

Boone's device is the result of classic biomedical engineering, combining mechanics, electrical systems, imaging technology, and high-speed computing. During the scan, which was being tested on human subjects in 2004 and 2005, the patient lies face down on a neoprene-like surface, her breast placed in an opening in the neoprene. The CT scanner then takes images of the breast from below the table—500 images in the prototype and eventually as many as 1,000 in later models. Boone and his assistants faced many challenges, including writing new algorithms and refining software to remove visual artifacts from the image.

"We pulled our hair," recalled Boone, 50. "We built the thing from scratch. But I'm a nerd. I like to build things."

He wound up using the equivalent of seventeen powerful personal computers, allowing him to scan a woman's breast in about fifteen seconds and produce a three-dimensional image in seven to ten minutes. Before scanning human subjects, he tested the accuracy of the scan on cadavers. One major advantage of Boone's breast scanner is that because the CT's X-ray beams are focused on a small object, the scan offers extremely detailed pictures while using less radiation. Boone's machine can spot tumors smaller than a pea, half the size of the tumors picked up reliably in a mammogram.

"We are virtually slicing and dicing the breast with this scanner," said Boone, the co-leader of the Biomedical Technology Program at the UC Davis Cancer Center. "The images are striking. A woman's prognosis is strongly linked to how small a tumor is when it's detected. Breast cancer has a 100-day doubling time, and if we can catch a tumor that's half the diameter, then that's equivalent to catching it almost a year earlier. As tumors grow larger, the chances of metastasis go up. The incidence of breast cancer increases with age, but the impact is greatest on middle-aged women. How many years are you taking away from people? Forty thousand women die a year from breast cancer, so if only 10 percent had a better survival rate because this CT scan works better than a mammogram, then at least 4,000 lives could be saved. It would be more expensive, but what is the ultimate expense of not detecting cancer early in the first place?"

All during the process, Boone, working closely with biomedical engineers at UC Davis and physicians at the cancer center, kept his eye on the ultimate goal: getting the scanner into clinical use.

"We are doing what the NIH is always talking about, which is translational research," said Boone. "We are taking a known technology and transferring it to a new application."

Katherine Ferrara's laboratory at UC Davis is doing the same thing with ultrasound technology. One of the most intriguing ultrasound research projects in Ferrara's lab is the use of "microbubbles," which are polymer or lipid bubbles—with a diameter about one-tenth that of a human hair—injected by the billions into a patient's bloodstream. The bubbles, which circulate safely in the cardiovascular system for several minutes before dissolving, have two major uses. First, they greatly enhance the quality of ultrasound images because the bubbling of the microspheres produces an ultrasound image with much more contrast and detail. They are already in clinical use in Europe as an ultrasound contrast agent.

Perhaps even more promising is the use of microbubbles to deliver drugs and genes, which could be attached to the outer shell of the microbubbles and then blasted into capillaries when the bubbles are zapped by ultrasound waves.

One promising technique would be to manufacture microbubbles with chemotherapy agents on the inside and antibodies on the outside designed to seek out certain enzymes or receptors on cancer cells. Once the microbubbles attached themselves to the cancer cell receptors, physicians could apply ultrasound to the area of the tumor and force the chemotherapy drug directly into the cancer cells. Doctors could dissolve blood clots in the heart or brain by using the ultrasound transducer to burst the bubbles and inject anticoagulant drugs directly into a clot. Studies also have shown that bursting microbubbles with ultrasound waves stimulates vessel growth, known as angiogenesis, which could give rise to treatments that would provide collateral circulation around areas of arterial blockage.

Graduate students in Ferrara's lab are investigating whether RNA—which takes genetic instructions from DNA and converts them into proteins—can be inserted into the nuclei of cells using microbubbles. Similar work is being undertaken at the University of Virginia by Dr. Jonathan Lindner, a cardiologist and proponent of microbubble research. Although delivering DNA with microbubbles is still in the early experimental stages, Lindner said it may be far safer than using viruses to implant disease-fighting DNA in cells. Bursting the microbubbles, he said, is like "using a grenade to blow DNA into a cell."

Another imaging frontier being explored at UC Davis is biomedical optics and photonics, which uses all kinds of light, from lasers to fluorescent light, to diagnose and treat disease. One of the most promising technologies is using lasers to determine whether cells are cancerous.

Stavros Demos, a physicist at the Lawrence Livermore National Laboratory and an investigator in the Center for Biophotonics at UC Davis, already has had considerable success detecting cancerous bladder lesions using light. The light is attached to the tip of a cystoscope, a thin, camera-tipped tube that can be inserted into the bladder through the urethra. By shining the laser on the inside of the bladder, Demos was able to identify cancer based on the way normal tissues and tumor tissues interact with laser light. His diagnoses turned out to be highly accurate based on samples taken from the bladder and later examined by a pathologist.

One day, surgeons might be able to use such a device to know instantly whether they have removed all cancer cells from the margins of tumors in the bladder, colon, esophagus, stomach, or skin.

"A cancer cell has increased metabolic activity, it's greedy and hungry and has a different look," said Dennis L. Matthews, director of the Center for Biophotonics. "Cancer cells have larger nuclei and more chromosomes. They're denser. All of this changes how light scatters off a cell. My question is, can we guide therapy? Can we help surgeons determine the margins? Can we do surgery at a single-cell level of precision? I've had neurosurgeons say, 'If you can do this, I can go in and remove a brain tumor without having to use chemotherapy and radiation. I can remove a tumor and not have to worry about it spreading.'"

At the University of Texas at Austin, biomedical engineering professor Rebecca Richards-Kortum has worked for more than a decade on a related technology to detect cervical cancer. In the procedure, known as fluorescence spectroscopy, a physician uses a fiber-optic probe to shine light on a patient's cervix, and the type and wavelength of the light that bounces off are analyzed by a computer. The technique relies on the same physical principle that Demos's laser scan employs, namely that cancer cells have a different structure than normal cells and absorb and refract light in a different way. Collaborating with Dr. Michele Follen, professor of gynecologic oncology at the University of Texas M. D. Anderson Cancer Center, Richards-Kortum is testing the probe on 1,800 patients. Preliminary results show that it is as accurate as conventional cervical cancer diagnostic techniques, which can be elaborate and result in a high percentage of false positives.

Richards-Kortum has estimated that her optical technique could save $625 million a year, result in far fewer false positives, and enable doctors to make earlier diagnoses of cervical cancer, which kills about 4,000 women in the United States annually. Her technology would be especially useful in developing countries, where rates of cervical cancer are far higher because of untreated gynecological diseases and where a lack of equipment and trained personnel makes it difficult to conduct even the most basic tests, such as a Pap smear. Cervical cancer is the second most prevalent cancer found in women worldwide and is the leading cancer killer among women in the developing world.

All these advances have made imaging a hot field, both for biomedical engineers and for radiologists, who were once relegated to a medical backwater. At the UC Davis Cancer Center, however, the greatest buzz today surrounds molecular imaging and molecular therapy, and doctors there are running numerous patient trials on targeted molecular cancer drugs and relying on molecular imaging to gauge their effectiveness.

One of those who participated in the trials and underwent molecular imaging was Aubrey C. Dixon. A retired general manager of a wholesale seed company near Fresno and a smoker from 1940 to 1980, Dixon developed a persistent cough in 2003 and was finally diagnosed in August of that year with lung cancer. An X-ray failed to show the tumor. But when Dixon, 76, was run through a PET scanner, the radioactive isotope FDG lit up his cancer, a clear example of the efficacy of molecular imaging. Based on the scan and other tests, doctors began treating Dixon with Taxol and carboplatin, two standard chemotherapy agents, which made him violently ill. He underwent thirty-four radiation treatments, tried another chemotherapy drug, and then heard about a trial being run by Dr. David Gandara of the UC Davis Cancer Center.

The trial involved a new drug called Tarceva, a targeted molecular agent that blocks a cancer cell protein, known as tyrosine kinase, which sends out signals for cancer cells to grow. The drug has shown some promise in shrinking non-small-cell tumors, the most common form of lung cancer and one that is very difficult to treat. Patients in Gandara's clinical trials have undergone conventional chemotherapy, which failed, and are hopeful that Tarceva might stave off the disease for months or years. All are aware, however, that cancer is a highly adaptive disease and that other targeted molecular agents—after an initial period of radical tumor shrinkage—have often been defeated by mutating cancer cells.

Throughout his therapy, Dixon was impressed with the accuracy of the four molecular PET images he received. They highlighted the cancer in his lung and also showed it spreading to his liver, where a small tumor had metastasized.

"These PET scans are absolutely marvelous," said Dixon. "The doctor sat down with us and showed us on the computer where all the new tumors were. . . . I was running out of options because the chemotherapy wasn't shrinking the tumors. Every test I had you could see it."

By the end of 2004, after four rounds of the new drug, the news was reasonably good. "The tumors are not growing," said Dixon. "They're holding their own."

The ordeal had caused Dixon's weight to seesaw, and when I met him, he weighed a respectable 156 pounds, down 20 pounds from his norm. An amiable, blue-eyed man with fair hair and oval glasses, Dixon was hospitalized when the initial dose of Tarceva proved too strong. He has been afflicted with rashes. Still, he was optimistic, or at least confident that he was receiving the best possible care that a cancer patient could receive at the start of the twenty-first century.

"There is no cure for lung cancer," said Dixon. "You have to be positive. You've got to get this thing done, or it's death."

When I said goodbye to Dixon and his wife of fifty-six years, Ernestine, I was hopeful that the new molecular therapy would give him many more months of life. He looked reasonably well and had a strong spirit. Only later did I discover that he died just ten days after our meeting. No one expected him to go so quickly, especially not his wife, who said goodnight to him as she did the dinner dishes and walked into the bedroom an hour later to find that his heart had given out under the weight of years of cancer.

Molecular imaging and targeted molecular drug therapy may one day save millions of lives. But for Aubrey Dixon, the new technology proved to be too little, too late.

Chapter 13

The Business

For more than two decades, Theodore Hersh was a professor of medicine at Emory University in Atlanta, living a full life of teaching and treating patients. In 1980, however, at the height of his career, Hersh—a gastroenterologist—noticed that his night vision, which had been poor for years, was getting worse. He also was losing the peripheral vision in his right eye. Visiting his ophthalmologist, Hersh learned that he had retinitis pigmentosa, a disease marked by the deterioration of the retina's photoreceptor cells, which pick up and process light signals sent to the brain. He quit driving in 1982, as the disease ate away at his peripheral vision and left him, particularly in the right eye, with the sensation that he was looking through a tunnel. Hersh continued teaching and practicing medicine until 1989, when, legally blind, he could no longer read X-rays well or master other small tasks of the job. His position as a professor was so intimately bound with his clinical work that he had to stop teaching, as well, a one-two blow that turned his world upside down.

"It was very hard for me, because I loved to see patients and I loved to teach," said Hersh, who also spent twenty-three years as chairman of Emory's Human Investigations Committee, which oversees clinical trials conducted at the university. "But having taken care of patients with so many illnesses and physical limitations, I knew I had to rise to the occasion and do the best I could. I was also fortunate to have the best partner in the world, my wife, and she has become my eyes."

Hersh continued working as an administrator at the Emory Clinic until 1995 and then founded a company with his wife, Rebecca, that manufactures antioxidant compounds and skin care products. Still, there was little he could do about the progression of his retinitis pigmentosa, a heretofore incurable disease, caused by various genetic mutations, that afflicts roughly 1 million people worldwide, many of them young and middle aged.

In late 2003, however, Hersh, then 70, was given some reason for hope, in the form of a tiny, fifteen-person biomedical engineering start-up company from Rhode Island. Driven by its resolute chief scientific officer, Weng Tao, the company—Neurotech—had overcome hurdle after hurdle before creating a potential treatment for people with retinitis pigmentosa and other degenerative retinal diseases. The therapy consists of a tiny device—about one-quarter of an inch long and as thin as pencil lead—inserted into the eye's gel-like vitreous humor and anchored to the wall of the eyeball. Inside the porous capsule are about 200,000 lab-grown human retinal cells that have been genetically modified to produce a protein called ciliary neurotrophic factor (CNTF) and release it slowly over time. Through years of research and many dead ends, Tao and Neurotech scientists had discovered that the device had the ability to stave off the death of retinal photoreceptors. Building on the work of two former Brown University scientists, they had worked out a method to keep the CNTF-producing cells alive in a capsule and implant that capsule inside the eye.

In short, Neurotech seemed to have achieved one of the great goals of twenty-first-century biomedical engineering: producing a cell-filled device—"a little factory to make protein," as Neurotech molecular biologist Paul Stabila put it—that could be implanted in the body to treat disease.

Experiments on specially bred dogs and rabbits with retinitis pigmentosa showed that the so-called encapsulated cell technology (ECT) slowed or halted the death of photoreceptor cells. And so, through the stubborn efforts of Tao and Neurotech vice president William Tente, the company was able to persuade the National Eye Institute—part of the National Institutes of Health—to conduct a limited trial of ten patients on the device's safety and efficacy. Hersh got wind of the trial, applied, met the qualifications to be included, and prepared to see whether somebody had finally come up with something to halt the progression of his retinitis pigmentosa, which will eventually leave him almost totally blind in both eyes. The physician who had overseen so many human trials was about to become a guinea pig himself.

"I spent so many years approving people to go into so many research studies," said Hersh. "People in these trials spent a lot of time helping us out in science and I said, 'This is my turn.'"

On June 9, 2004, Hersh traveled with his wife to Bethesda, Maryland, where an eye surgeon, in a fifteen-minute operation, implanted the minuscule device into Hersh's right eye.

Just a few weeks before, across the country in California, a young boy was taking part in another clinical trial. This one also consisted of ten people, all children with Type 1 diabetes, and also involved a device—a pump that checked the children's glucose levels every five minutes and delivered insulin into their bloodstream to regulate their blood sugar levels. There, however, the similarities ended, for the company involved in the California trial was not a fifteen-person start-up that had burned through tens of millions of dollars and never earned a penny of revenue. The company was Medtronic, and if ever a David and Goliath comparison was apt, this was it.

Medtronic is the oldest and largest of all the world's biomedical engineering companies, a multinational behemoth that in 2004 employed 32,000 people and sold more than $9 billion worth of medical devices in 120 countries. Half a century earlier, the company had gotten its start making heart pacemakers, but over the decades—through aggressive research and development, marketing, and acquisitions—it had become involved in just about every aspect of medical technology. Medtronic made heart defibrillators. It made heart valves. It made stents to prop open clogged arteries. It made devices to fuse spinal vertebrae and implantable pumps to dull pain. It made equipment to perform brain surgery and electrical brain stimulators to quiet the tremors of people with Parkinson's disease. And it made several devices—from pumps to tiny computers that calculate insulin doses—to treat diabetes, one of the fastest-growing diseases in America.

In the 2004 California trial, Medtronic was testing a new piece of diabetes wizardry, and Jennifer and Rick Caughman—along with their 10-year-old diabetic son, Tim—wanted Tim to have a crack at the next big thing to come through the company's pipeline. Tim and his parents already were enjoying the latest commercially available diabetes-fighting technology from Medtronic. It was an external pump, about the size of a pager, that dispensed a baseline amount of insulin to Tim through a small, disposable tube attached to his abdomen. When Tim ate a meal or a snack, he or his parents entered the number of carbohydrates into the pump, which calculated how much insulin he needed to metabolize the extra glucose in his system. In addition, the Medtronic pump system contained a computerized meter that would read Tim's blood sugar levels, based on a finger-stick, and automatically transmit those readings to the pump unit on Tim's belt.

Tim was originally diagnosed with diabetes in June 2000, an event that sent the family into upheaval as they struggled to manage his diet, his wildly fluctuating blood sugars, and his insulin shots. Two events restored a sense of normalcy and peace to the Caughman family: coming under the care of the renowned juvenile diabetes program at the Childrens Hospital Los Angeles, and getting a Medtronic insulin pump in April 2001. The pump eliminated the need both for rigidly calculating what Tim ate and when, and for giving him frequent insulin injections.

"Before and after the pump was like night and day," said Jennifer Caughman. "It changed everything."

But Medtronic had further improved its insulin pump system and in the spring of 2004 offered the Caughmans the chance to bring Tim into a one-month trial. The new device, known as the Paradigm REAL-time Insulin Pump and Continuous Glucose Monitoring System, offered two significant advances over the pump Tim was using. First, a glucose sensor implanted under the skin of his abdomen continuously transmitted his glucose levels to the pump. Second, the new sensor-augmented pump gave Tim's parents a constantly updated trend graph of his blood sugar levels, helping them know whether his glucose levels were changing and, if so, in what direction. This was a vital tool in effectively matching the amount of insulin he receives with the amount of glucose in his blood. (Insulin, in effect, escorts glucose into cells, where it can be metabolized.) Both of these advances would enable Tim and his parents to control his diabetes even more closely, which is the key to preventing the onset of the devastating consequences of the disease. These can include cardiovascular disease, kidney failure, blindness, and damage to nerves and vessels in the foot, which sometimes leads to amputation.

So in April 2004, just as Hersh was preparing to try out Neurotech's encapsulated cell technology for his retinitis pigmentosa, Tim was poised to receive the latest diabetes-busting device to be invented by Medtronic MiniMed engineers. The Caughmans knew that this newest pump was just another step along a road that would eventually lead to what Medtronic calls its artificial pancreas—a fully implantable system in which sensors inside the body relay information to a pump, which is also inside the body. The pump then automatically calculates and delivers the precise amount of insulin a person requires to normalize blood sugar levels.

But that day could wait. For now, the Caughmans were thrilled that Tim was about to test-drive the latest model of the pump.

"These pumps give you more freedom and flexibility," said Tim's father, Rick Caughman, a commercial artist. "They give you more peace of mind. They give you a better sense of what's going on. And this technology allows kids to be kids. The bottom line is that this technology has given my kid a childhood. It frees him up to go about his life. My kid does kung fu. My kid does roller blades. That's the net result."

Two patients. Two companies. Together, the stories of Medtronic and Neurotech tell the tale of the business of biomedical engineering, which, in half a century, has gone from a handful of companies making X-ray machines and hospital equipment to a sprawling industry at the cutting edge of medicine and health care. The rise of Medtronic, launched in 1949 by electrical engineer Earl Bakken and his brother-in-law in a Minneapolis garage, is the symbol of the ascension of the medical technology industry in America and around the world. But as successful as it is, Medtronic is only one of a host of major companies now flourishing in the realm of biomedical engineering and biotechnology. Boston Scientific, St. Jude Medical, Guidant, Johnson & Johnson, General Electric, Siemens—these and other companies are contributing to rapid improvements in global health care and steadily increasing life expectancy in developed countries. They are joined by biotechnology firms like Genentech, Amgen, and Genzyme, which produce everything from chemotherapy agents to insulin for diabetics.

All these businesses—from traditional device makers, to imaging companies, to firms on the cutting edge of genetic and biological research—are reshaping and renewing the American commercial landscape. At a time when traditional American heavy industry and manufacturing are disappearing in the face of intense foreign competition, high-tech biomedical firms are stepping in to fill the void. I witnessed this transformation in places like Pittsburgh, where the steel mills that once lined the Monongahela River are being torn down and replaced by sleek, low-rise offices housing medical and bioengineering companies. Much of this growth is associated with the intellectual capital found at nearby institutions like the University of Pittsburgh and Carnegie Mellon. In Atlanta, biomedical engineering and health care research taking place at Georgia Tech and Emory is a magnet for biotechnology businesses. In Minnesota, a cluster of companies started by former Medtronic employees—including St. Jude and Guidant—has played an integral role in the creation of the corridor known as Medical Alley, which stretches from Rochester, Minnesota, home of the Mayo Clinic, to the Twin Cities and farther north. An estimated 250,000 people are now employed in the biomedical firms, hospitals, and universities that make up Minnesota's Medical Alley.

And then there are the start-ups, such as Neurotech, hoping to emerge from obscurity and bring products to the public. Whether Neurotech's encapsulated cell technology for retinal diseases—which affect 50 million people worldwide—ever makes it to market is an open question. But in some ways, the story of Neurotech's struggle to stay alive and pioneer new biomedical engineering technology has parallels to the early days of Medtronic. Both certainly had modest beginnings. Indeed, when Earl Bakken and his brother-in-law, Palmer Hermundslie, launched Medtronic, they worked out of a 600-square-foot garage that they heated in winter with a pot-bellied stove and cooled in summer by spraying water on the roof. In their first month of operation, they racked up total net sales of $8 for repairing a centrifuge. At one point in its early years, the company even faced insolvency.

The greatest parallel between Medtronic and Neurotech, however, is the drive and vision of Bakken and Tao, Neurotech's chief scientific officer. Over the past decade, Tao also has faced huge problems and yanked her vision of encapsulated cell technology out of the ashes on several occasions. Her co-workers affectionately describe her as a "bulldog" or a "pit bull" and unanimously agree that without her grit the enterprise would be dead.

When Tao's colleagues talk about her and their lean organization, their descriptions echo the words Bakken wrote in 1979 when he described the qualities needed to invent and produce a successful medical device. The creator, wrote Bakken, should be "devoted to his idea [device] helping someone, not simply being a commercial success. . . . Always a very small number on team. Usually non-conformist, a strong missionary zeal for the idea. . . . Has great persistence in the face of great criticism. Great persuasion or coercion to get the idea accepted . . . a maverick, a risk taker . . . oblivious to criticism."

To all who know her, it sounds like Weng Tao.

"We've been through hell several times and bounced back," Tao told me when I visited Neurotech's offices in Lincoln, Rhode Island, 12 miles north of Providence. "I don't take no for an answer. I learned that if you have a vision and want to realize that vision, you can do that, no matter what."

Nine days before Christmas 2003, on a cold, clear afternoon, Earl Bakken stood before 231 Medtronic employees in a small auditorium just off the soaring, glass-enclosed atrium at the company's world headquarters in Minneapolis. Bakken was dressed in charcoal gray pants, a navy blue blazer, and a pink and green Hawaiian shirt—a flourish acknowledging the state he now calls home. He was accompanied by a nurse, for at age 81, Bakken—though mentally sharp—is suffering from diabetes and cardiovascular disease. Indeed, Bakken, as he would shortly point out to the group, is a walking advertisement for Medtronic products. One of the corporation's pacemakers regulates his heart, a Medtronic diabetes pump supplies him with insulin, and an artery is propped open with a company stent. As he waited to speak, Bakken looked the antithesis of the driven American mogul, and with good reason; although undeniably wealthy, he never aspired to be a baron of industry. He was an engineer and an inventor, and his demeanor is gentle and grandfatherly. His hair is light brown with touches of gray, his eyes blue, his face is round and adorned with a pair of large, wire-rimmed glasses, and his gait is slow, a result of nerve damage to his feet from diabetes.

That day, as he has every year for decades, Bakken was presiding over a Medtronic "Mission and Medallion Ceremony," a ritual in which he greets new employees. In few megacorporations today does the founder shake hands with every beginning worker, but Bakken still does, hewing to a ritual that says something about Medtronic's corporate culture. Scientists and other employees there are still inspired by the company's mission—to save and improve lives through biomedical engineering—and Bakken insists on imparting that message in person. He is fond of noting that every six seconds someone in the world is treated with a Medtronic product. The corporate logo shows a patient rising from a table to a standing position. "Medtronic," the logo reads. "Where Life Depends on Medical Technology."

The audience of young, well-dressed employees sat silently as Bakken recounted the history of the company he had created and they had joined. He told them how he saw the movie *Frankenstein* in 1932 and knew then that he wanted "to use electricity to reanimate man."

He described the genesis of Medtronic, which began when Bakken—an electrical engineer—was hanging around the hospital where his wife worked as a medical technologist and doctors started asking him to repair equipment. He described the early turning point in the company's life: the close collaboration with legendary heart surgeon C. Walton Lillehei to develop the first transistorized pacemakers. That moment, Bakken recalled, came in October 1957, when Lillehei was performing operations on so-called blue babies, whose skin color had a blue hue because a heart defect left them with too little oxygenated blood. Lillehei, at the University of Minnesota, successfully operated on the children to repair the defect. But about 20 percent experienced postoperative "heart block," a condition in which the surgery interfered with the conduction of electricity through the cardiac muscle. A large external pacemaker, the size of a television and powered by AC current, had been invented by Paul M. Zoll in Boston. Lillehei helped reduce the power of the machine for use in children, but on October 31, 1957, during a three-hour power blackout, the pacemakers being used by several "heart block" children stopped running. One of them died.

To prevent another needless death, Lillehei asked Bakken to devise a battery-powered pacemaker. Displaying the ingenuity that was the hallmark of early biomedical engineering, Bakken cobbled together a pacemaker by copying the circuitry from an electric metronome described in *Popular Electronics* magazine. He scavenged parts from other devices in his garage workshop and hooked up the pacemaker—which consisted of a 4-inch-square body with wires running into the chest—to a 9-volt battery. The entire process took a month. He tested the device in a dog, and it worked.

"The next day I went to the university and saw this attached to a child's body," Bakken told the group, holding up one of the original pacemakers. "That was quite an experience because something we had made with our own hands was keeping this child alive. This really opened up the world to pacing. We didn't have any idea of the revolution we would start."

In his soft, flat Minnesota accent, Bakken told the gathering that the swiftness with which the first battery-powered pacemaker was designed, built, and used on patients was the best example of one of his axioms: "Ready. Fire. Aim." By that he meant that rather than studying things to death, biomedical engineers had to keep in mind the goal of getting devices to patients, even if all the kinks had not been removed. What he did not state—but pointed out in a later interview—is that in an age of long trials and intense regulation by the FDA, that command is now far more difficult to execute.

"People said Medtronic wanted your heart," Bakken told the assembly. "Now we want every part of your body. The whole body is electric. Our work restores a person to a full flesh and blood human being. People come up to me and say, 'Mr. Bakken, you have given me my life back.' But it's really you"—Bakken gestured toward his audience—"that have given them their life back. . . . This mission statement is not just something posted on the door. It's something we live by. I want to emphasize that this is *your* mission, to play a role helping people to a better, fuller life."

After Medtronic's chairman and CEO, Arthur D. Collins Jr., addressed the gathering, Bakken was escorted to the side of the stage, where he shook the hands of the new employees and handed each of them a Medtronic medallion. Several dozen workers asked to be photographed with the legendary founder, and Bakken complied, smiling with each flash. He may have been unassuming and a bit frail, but he was the star of the show, a living piece of history whose venture, born in a garage, went on to improve health care around the globe.

Under Bakken's leadership, Medtronic grew steadily from the 1950s to the 1970s, its identity built around cardiac pacemakers, widely considered one of the top medical inventions of the twentieth century. The company's engineers continually refined the pacemaker to make it smaller, more reliable, and more responsive to a patient's demand, which meant that when a patient exercised, the pacemaker would increase its number of beats. Paul Citron, an engineer who joined the company in 1972 and rose to be vice president of Science and Technology before retiring in 2003, said Bakken's influence permeated Medtronic, fostering a wide-open, practical research effort that led to innovation and success.

"The attitude was, 'Yes, you have a job to do, but let's leave you some flexibility to innovate,'" said Citron, who did groundbreaking work on anchoring pacemaker leads in the heart. "The other thing about Earl was that he had a very small ego. He created a system that gave a high level of credit to his employees."

Bakken also had a clear idea of what constituted a successful medical device, and he was careful not to pursue wild-eyed schemes, according to Citron and others. To succeed, Bakken said a device had to meet certain criteria. It had to be implantable. It had to address a long-standing, unmet medical need. There had to be no other alternatives to the device, and it had to provide rapid, noticeable improvement to the patient. It also had to operate on its own, without the patient worrying much about maintenance.

Despite sales growth of 15 to 20 percent a year and the entry of Medtronic into other businesses, such as heart valves, the company hit a rough patch in the late 1970s and early 1980s. A line of pacemakers had to be recalled because some failed after body fluids leaked inside. Bakken began easing out of the day-to-day operations of the company, stepping down as CEO in 1976. And by the early 1980s, the company had become "pretty fat, dumb, and happy," recalled Citron, its share of the pacemaker market plunging from 64 percent in 1972 to 28 percent in 1986. Other companies, such as St. Jude, were cutting into Medtronic's market with aggressive sales techniques, and the company's research and development operation had lost its edge. The turnaround began in 1985 when a new CEO, Winston R. Wallin, restructured the company. Medtronic's recovery hit full stride in 1989 with the arrival of William W. (Bill) George as president and later CEO. He oversaw a period of acquisitions that led the company into a host of new device businesses, most notably the acquisition of the diabetes device company, MiniMed, in 2001 for $3.8 billion.

Today, Medtronic has fought its way back to a preeminent position in the pacemaker business, selling nearly half of the roughly 1 million pacemakers placed annually in people worldwide. It makes half of the 200,000 defibrillators sold every year in the United States.

Medtronic also dominates the diabetes device business, having sold more than 70 percent of the 300,000 insulin pumps now used in America. In addition, Medtronic has expanded aggressively into the spinal surgery and spinal fusion business, into control of chronic pain with electrical stimulation and drug-dispensing pumps, and into electrical stimulation of the brain to quiet the tremors of Parkinson's disease and other movement disorders.

Like the entire field of biomedical engineering, the company is expanding its horizons beyond devices and into the world of biology and genetics. In fact, tiny Neurotech and gargantuan Medtronic are now pursuing research in a common field—"convergence" devices, which combine traditional biomedical engineering devices with cellular therapies.

These days, Bakken devotes much of his time to establishing what he calls "high-tech, high-touch" hospitals in Hawaii and in other states, combining the latest medical advances with traditional healing. He continues to stay abreast of developments in biomedical engineering and health care, subscribing to 178 journals and magazines.

"You've got to move so fast in this field now," Bakken, wearing a "Pray for Peace" button and an American flag pin, said in an interview. "It's just not the same as it used to be. Two-thirds of our income is from products that we have brought to market in the last two years."

Nowhere is that innovation more clearly on display than in Medtronic's Cardiac Rhythm Management division, the mainstay of its business, accounting for nearly half of its annual revenues. Citron describes the evolution of cardiac devices as "taking a Model T and turning it into a Lexus," with pacemakers today doing a lot more than driving sluggish hearts. In its new three-lead, triple-chamber iteration, the device can so precisely synchronize the heartbeat that it creates a more efficient pumping action for people in heart failure.

Improvements in defibrillators have been equally impressive, as Medtronic engineers attempt to combat a condition—sudden cardiac arrest—that kills roughly 400,000 Americans a year. (Sudden cardiac arrest typically occurs because of fibrillation.) The roots of defibrillation technology reach back more than two centuries, as doctors and scientists experimented with restarting dog and human hearts by applying an electrical charge. But it wasn't until 1970 that Dr. Michael Mirowski of the Johns Hopkins University successfully developed and implanted the first defibrillator in a human. Today, defibrillators are a $2 billion business for Medtronic, and the room for growth is sizable. Millions of people at risk for ventricular fibrillation still do not have the devices, and Medtronic executives believe the company's defibrillator sales could triple or quadruple in the coming years.

Much of the early defibrillator research conducted by Medtronic scientists in the late 1980s and early 1990s was classic biomedical engineering that focused on two areas. The first was reducing the device from a baseball-sized apparatus that fit into the abdomen, with wires running to the heart, to a watch-sized machine implanted easily into the hollow of the shoulder. The second focus was on continuing to improve the formulas and algorithms that could distinguish between benign heartbeats that were rapid or irregular—occurring, say, during exercise—and fibrillation.

Medtronic engineers have now invented a so-called pain-free defibrillator feature that eliminates many extraneous shocks by first using pacemaker technology to try to "pace" the heart out of rapid beating and only as a last resort zapping the patient with a shock. The shocks are brief but powerful, and patients describe being blasted out of their chairs or being knocked over by the charge. With older devices, patients sometimes receive unneeded shocks, severely diminishing their ardor for the defibrillator.

"You can go back and forth about whether a 400-volt shock is painful or startling, but the point is you'll get very little argument about whether you want an unnecessary shock," said Paul Belk, a Medtronic researcher who received a Ph.D. from the Harvard-MIT Health Sciences and Technology Program. "Of all the shocks given for fibrillation, many were unnecessary. It's very disturbing. It's very unpleasant, and we know some patients who get multiple shocks and barricade themselves in the bedroom. It's a huge problem and one we have to solve."

Engineers such as Paul DeGroot have done a computer analysis of thousands of fibrillation records to help them create a machine that better identifies true fibrillation. If the device senses that the heart is indeed descending into fibrillation—a process it identifies in six seconds—it begins administering a series of strong but imperceptible charges. If that pacing fails to halt fibrillation in fifteen to twenty seconds, the device administers a strong shock. Clinical studies have shown that pacing the heart out of defibrillation works in about three-quarters of cases, drastically reducing the number of shocks.

"If we could cut the number of shocks in half, we could make a big difference to a lot of people," said Belk.

The engineers doing defibrillator research have deep backgrounds in medicine and engineering. Rob Stadler, who also has a Ph.D. from the Harvard-MIT Health Sciences and Technology Program, spent a year at Harvard Medical School, often accompanying doctors on their rounds at Brigham and Women's Hospital. The experience gave him insight into the needs of doctors and the still great demand for better devices and medical technology.

"It changed my whole perspective," said Stadler, whose Ph.D. is in medical engineering. "I did hospital rounds for half a year. I met a patient with a defibrillator who went skiing and got his heart rate up and got a big shock that dropped him to his knees. I thought, 'How stupid! Someone goes skiing and they got a shock. I'd like to do something about that.'

"Another time there was this big discussion about a heart failure patient and they were trying to assess her fluid status. I was just amazed at how subjective it was. I carried a little notebook around with me and I had a section called 'Big Unmet Medical Needs' and I wrote these things in there. And here I've been working on these devices that have enhanced our ability to avoid unnecessary shocks or identify when fluid is building up in someone."

DeGroot is hopeful that biomedical advances will eventually render the defibrillator obsolete. One possibility, he said, is to develop a pacemaker that would actually prevent the heart from going into fibrillation. Another alternative would be a molecular or cellular therapy to replace the damaged cardiac tissue that causes fibrillation.

"We don't just want to make a better shock box, we want to prevent the underlying condition from developing," said DeGroot. "We want to cure the problem."

It was inevitable that Medtronic would find its way into the diabetes-fighting business, for few diseases pose more of a threat to America's overall health and can be as effectively treated with a medical device. Medtronic's entry into the field came in 2000 with the acquisition of the insulin pump maker MiniMed, and since then Medtronic has used its extensive research and development (R&D) capabilities—the company spends about $850 million a year on R&D—and its international sales network to establish a dominant position in the insulin pump market.

An estimated 20 million people in the United States now have diabetes. Roughly 1.3 million of those have Type 1 diabetes, also known as juvenile diabetes. Type 1 diabetes usually strikes people at a young age and is caused by an autoimmune reaction in which the body attacks and destroys insulin-making cells in the pancreas. All people with Type 1 diabetes are dependent on insulin, and more than 20 percent use an insulin pump.

But by far the largest number of diabetics in the country have Type 2 diabetes, many of whom have come down with the disease because they are part of the growing army of obese people in the United States. More than 18 million Americans now have Type 2 diabetes, 13 million of whom have been diagnosed with the disease and 5 million of whom still don't know they have the condition. Over time, people with Type 2 diabetes become dependent on insulin, and today about 2.7 million Americans with Type 2 diabetes use insulin. Only a fraction of those, however—less than 2 percent—are on the insulin pump, meaning their diabetes is often not well controlled. Failing to keep blood sugar levels under tight control can shorten diabetics' lives by a decade or more, as they are prone to a host of complications. Health care officials have estimated that the cost of treating diabetes in the United States is currently $130 billion a year.

"Many people don't understand the impact diabetes is having on our country," said Robert Guezuraga, president of Medtronic Diabetes. "If trends continue, one out of three people in the U.S. could get diabetes."

Guezuraga is, of course, a proponent of the insulin pump and estimates that sales for Medtronic MiniMed will increase by 18 to 24 percent a year for the next five years. But even those without a financial interest in selling insulin pumps agree that it is the best technology available to treat insulin-dependent diabetics. (Many Type 2 diabetics can bring their disease under control without insulin if they lose weight, follow a restricted diet, and exercise.) Clinical trials have shown that users of the pump, which can release pinhead-sized amounts of insulin inside the body, have significantly fewer complications than diabetics who more loosely control their disease.

Medtronic executives don't need to sell pump users on the device. The vast majority of diabetics who have tried the pump are fervent devotees of the technology. To many families like the Caughmans whose children have developed Type 1 diabetes, the pump often was the turning point in their fight against the disease.

Tim Caughman's diabetes came on with alarming swiftness. Over the course of several days, when he was just 6 years old, Tim was suddenly hit with a desperate thirst and the need to urinate constantly. On the night of June 14, 2000, the Caughmans—who live in Ontario, California, not far from Los Angeles—put Tim to bed at 8 p.m. By 2 a.m. he had gotten up to urinate nine times. His parents knew then that something was wrong, and the next morning Jennifer Caughman made an emergency appointment with Tim's pediatrician. But before heading to the doctor's office, she had time to get on the Internet, and within a few minutes she knew that Tim had diabetes. Urine and blood tests at the pediatrician's office confirmed her fears.

The next few days were a blur, as the Caughmans put their sick son in the hospital for three days and doctors struggled to bring his sharply vacillating blood sugar under control.

"It was incredible, the whole thing was overwhelming," said Jennifer Caughman, an administrator at Scripps College in Claremont,

California. "We basically had to get a degree in biology in two days. The information they pass on to you to manage your child's life is overwhelming. It is a very humbling disease. It is very unpredictable. It turned us into absolute idiots overnight. We didn't know what to do for the kid or how to keep him comfortable, healthy and safe. It was pretty bleak."

Frustrated by the quality of care they were receiving locally, the Caughmans eventually went to Childrens Hospital Los Angeles, where Tim was treated by one of the country's leading experts in diabetes, Dr. Francine R. Kaufmann. Under her care, the Caughmans slashed Tim's insulin doses by 75 percent and brought his blood sugar levels into a safe range. Kaufmann said the insulin pump would be a good solution for Tim, and after a few months the Caughmans were more than ready to try one. Even under the best possible care and with two parents who learned as much as they could about the disease, managing Tim's diabetes was an ordeal. He had to eat a tightly controlled diet at rigidly prescribed times and receive several insulin shots a day. Even then, anything from a cold, to exercise, to fatigue could cause his blood sugar levels to soar or plunge.

The Medtronic pump smoothed out that rocky road. The device delivered a small, steady supply of insulin into Tim's system, known as the basal dose, and whenever he ate, the family could plug the meal's carbohydrate count into the pump's computer, which would calculate the additional insulin, or bolus, he needed. Every few days the Caughmans would refill the insulin reservoir in the pump, which was attached to Tim's belt and fed insulin into his system through a catheter in his abdomen.

"Two big things changed when we started using the pump," Jennifer Caughman told me in a phone interview. "One is that Tim could eat whatever he wanted whenever he wanted it. He could skip dinner. He could sleep in because the basal rate keeps his blood sugar normal without food. We're not on a diabetes schedule anymore. That was an incredible intrusion into our lives."

"The bottom line," Rick Caughman said in the background, "is that Tim is a healthier and happier kid."

"We're all healthier and happier," said Jennifer. "And the second wonderful thing now is that his diabetes is under such tight control. If you tried to do that kind of tight control with shots, you'd be going through ten syringes a day, and his arm would be a pincushion."

The trial of the new device—which featured a disposable glucose sensor implanted inside Tim and a trend graph of his blood sugar levels—brought even more control over his disease and greater peace of mind to the family.

"Tim could be in class and pull out his device and it would tell him, 'Right now, your blood sugar is 85,' and it would show him if it was going up or dropping," said Jennifer Caughman. "He could look and say, 'I'm going low soon, I'm going to have some juice.' It's an amazing thing. Tim called it the 'Gizmo.' We always knew where his blood sugar was and where it was heading."

At night, Rick Caughman no longer had to get up once or twice to stick Tim's finger and check his blood sugar. Instead, he would get up once and look at the device, which showed him Tim's glucose trends, and usually go back to sleep assured that his son would be fine for the night.

The trial pump also contained voluminous information about Tim's blood sugar levels, which nurses and doctors at Childrens Hospital could download to a computer and analyze. Using that data, they changed the baseline insulin rate he was receiving. Such interactive equipment is part of a trend at Medtronic to produce devices, including pacemakers and defibrillators, that store data for physicians and nurses to gain access to in the office or over the Internet. The company's CareLink Network now enables more than 130,000 patients with cardiac rhythm devices to transmit data from their devices to physicians over the phone or the Internet.

The trial, which included Tim and nine other children, ended in April 2004. The results were generally good, and Medtronic was planning to bring the sensor-augmented pump to market by early 2006—a date the Caughmans are anxiously awaiting.

"We almost fled the country to keep it," said Jennifer Caughman. "It was an incredible piece of equipment. We're just dying for this thing to come back. It gave us so much information, and it gave Tim a lot of confidence."

The insulin pump also has given Jennifer and Rick Caughman the confidence that their son will defy the traditional odds that a child with diabetes will, on average, live eighteen fewer years than a non-diabetic child.

"I have no doubt that he will have a long, healthy life," said Jennifer Caughman. "With the technology he has now, he has the tools he needs."

Indeed, the technology available to Tim Caughman will only get better. Medtronic and other companies are working toward the creation of an "artificial pancreas." Medtronic is developing two versions, one external and one implantable. The implantable model would feature a glucose sensor that would relay information to an implantable pump, which would then automatically deliver insulin to a patient's blood. Fourteen patients in France and six in California are already experimenting with an early version of this system, which could eventually remove nearly all the thought and labor that diabetics must now devote to their disease.

Some companies are eyeing an even more futuristic therapy, not unlike Neurotech's encapsulated cell technology. In this scenario, cells that could sense glucose and produce insulin would be encased in a small device implanted in a person's abdomen, essentially taking over the function of a diseased pancreas. No pumps, no mechanical sensors, just cells in a device that acts like a human organ. It may seem far-fetched, but already Medtronic, like its competitors, is working on ways to marry traditional biomedical engineering devices with a new universe of cellular and genetic therapies.

The buzzword for this emerging technology is "convergence device," and research into this union of machines and cells takes place in the laboratories of the Materials and Biosciences Center at Medtronic's Minneapolis headquarters. There, engineers, biochemists, physicians, and cellular and molecular biologists are investigating ways to lead the company into another realm. Spearheading these efforts are two women: Rebecca Bergman, Medtronic's vice president for Science and Technology, and Maura Donovan, the senior director of Biosciences Research and Development.

Medtronic's move into "convergence" technology reflects a wider trend transforming biomedical engineering. Long the domain of engineers and physicians who invented machines and devices to treat patients, the field is now exploring the most exciting scientific frontier of our time—human genetics and cellular and molecular biology. No one at Medtronic would suggest that devices are on their way out, but a growing understanding exists that genetics and cellular therapies may one day offer cures for conditions that devices can now only treat.

"There has been an explosion of knowledge in the life sciences, and the convergence of life sciences and medical devices is a growing area of interest for Medtronic," said Bergman, who was trained as a chemical engineer.

Said Donovan, who has a Ph.D. in pharmacology, "Devices have been tremendously successful for Medtronic. What we're looking at is where can biology add to devices and how can biology take us where devices may not take us? How do biology and devices work together to enhance each other?"

Medtronic has already taken some first steps in the direction of convergence devices. The company now coats many pacemaker leads with a steroid-releasing substance, which improves their longevity by minimizing the buildup of scar tissue around the electrode. The company also has a combination product used in patients who undergo spinal fusion to treat degenerative disk disease. Medtronic impregnates a collagen sponge with a human growth factor that stimulates bone growth to help fuse the two levels of the spine.

In 2004 and 2005, Medtronic announced several collaborations that propelled it farther down the path of bringing biology and genetics into the company's core device business. Medtronic and the Massachusetts-based biotechnology company Genzyme have established a joint venture to investigate whether cells derived from a person's thigh muscle can be injected into heart muscle damaged in heart attacks, possibly regenerating the area of damaged tissue. In the procedure, currently being tried in some patients in Europe, the muscle cells are harvested, expanded in culture, and injected into the patient's diseased cardiac tissue during a heart bypass operation. Skeletal muscle cells have a greater potential to regenerate than heart muscle cells, and scientists are investigating whether a method can be found to insert the cells and have them take over some of the function of the damaged cells. Genzyme and Medtronic also are investigating ways to genetically modify the skeletal muscle cells to improve their performance as heart tissue.

"If you find a biological way to have the heart regrow cells and reestablish its own pacemaker, that would be the Holy Grail," said Bergman. "Is that likely in our lifetime? I don't know."

A potentially more ambitious project involves the use of biological therapies to treat neurodegenerative diseases such as Alzheimer's and Parkinson's. Medtronic and a Massachusetts-based biotech firm, Alnylam Pharmaceuticals, are collaborating on a therapy—known as RNA interference therapy (RNAi)—designed to block the production of proteins that play a role in these afflictions. The goal of RNAi is to intervene in the process by which DNA sends signals to RNA, thus inhibiting the production of certain proteins. Alnylam will focus on the genetic aspects of the therapy, and Medtronic will concentrate on developing a way to deliver the RNAi to the affected portions of the brain. One way of delivering the therapy might be a small, implantable pump that would continually release molecules to obstruct the production of the tangled plaques that cause Alzheimer's or the pathogens that kill dopamine cells in people with Parkinson's.

Around Medtronic, many engineers are intrigued by the company's foray into the brave new world of genetics and cellular biology but unworried that this will soften the focus on the devices that have made Medtronic what it is today.

"I'm okay with not riding the big wave into the next big thing," said Paul Belk of Cardiac Rhythm Management. "You can ask if those of us who work with wires and electrodes and solid state circuits wake up in a cold sweat worrying that we will be dinosaurs. People challenge me, 'Aren't you going to be out of date soon?' I might be. But the work we do is important and needs improvement. There are a ton of people walking around with electrical therapy devices like pacemakers for ten, fifteen, twenty years. When biotech gets a track record like that, come and talk to me."

CHAPTER 14

Weng's Wars

In her struggle to find a treatment for debilitating eye diseases like retinitis pigmentosa, Weng Tao has faced innumerable woes. Fortunately for her and her colleagues at the biomedical start-up Neurotech, Tao also has possessed an equal measure of single-minded drive. As a result, the tiny Neurotech team has done what few small companies ever accomplish: getting a product into human clinical trials. Tao and her colleagues also are tantalizingly close to combining cellular therapies with a device, an elusive goal in the world of biomedical engineering. None of this would likely have happened without Tao, whose self-assurance and resourcefulness were forged in her early years in China.

Tao was born in Beijing in 1959. As a girl she lived through a decade of repression during Mao Zedong's Cultural Revolution and entered university a year after Mao's death in 1976. She eventually went to medical school and worked for a year as an intern in Beijing Childrens Hospital.

"Basically I felt very helpless when I was told there were no treatments for many life-threatening diseases," said Tao, an unassuming, plainspoken woman with black hair cut neatly to her chin. "I saw patients die under my care. I saw children die. A doctor can't help patients if there is no effective therapy for a disease. And I realized that maybe being an MD was not good enough for me. So I thought maybe I should go into a field where I can design new therapies."

While living in China, she learned to maneuver within a hostile system, a skill that would serve her well when the atmosphere turned chilly and discordant in some of the companies that preceded Neurotech.

"In China for me to do anything at all I had to be very creative or I'd wind up trapped in bureaucracy," said Tao. "I could see that the U.S. was the land of opportunity. But when I got here I found that many people believe things can't be done because there are so many rules and regulations. People have the opportunities but often they choose not to explore them. People would tell me that the FDA would never allow us to use the cells we chose for the encapsulated cell technology [ECT], but I would say, 'Rules are made by people. Let's show them the data and persuade them to change their positions.' I often ask questions and negotiate a solution. I don't necessarily just accept the answers."

Tao came to the United States in 1983 at age 24, receiving a Ph.D. in cell physiology and biophysics at the University of Connecticut Health Center. She went on to do postdoctoral research in molecular immunology at Yale University and then worked for several companies. In 1996 she went to work for a Rhode Island biotechnology start-up, CytoTherapeutics. Among the company's endeavors was an effort to commercialize an encapsulated cell technology developed by two Swiss scientists, Patrick Aebischer and Pier Galletti, both then of Brown University. The pair invented one of the earliest versions of the technology, which involved, in Tao's words, "loading cells that produce a therapeutic factor in a capsule, which is implanted in a host." The goal was to treat diseases such as diabetes and Parkinson's with a long-lasting stream of substances, such as insulin or dopamine, generated by cells inside the permeable capsule. From the beginning, however, scientists at CytoTherapeutics faced an overwhelming challenge: how to ensure that the cells, encased in a semipermeable membrane, stayed alive and churned out disease-fighting molecules.

The company, which at one point had more than a hundred employees, dropped the diabetes research early on. The Parkinson's experiments met the same fate. The company did conduct human trials on a device filled with cells that released a pain-killing substance, but results in clinical trials showed it to have marginal effect.

Meanwhile, Tao was deep into research she believed showed great promise—genetically modifying encapsulated cells to secrete therapeutic proteins. She continued to work on numerous scientific challenges, including keeping the cells alive for an extended period of time in the capsule. But as she delved deeper into her work, CytoTherapeutics plunged into financial trouble, and the environment became increasingly "toxic," according to molecular biologist Paul Stabila, one of Tao's colleagues. Tao said she was discouraged from spending more money and time on finding a suitable cell line for ECT.

"Basically I was told to mind my own business," said Tao. "The top people told me, 'You'll never find cells that live in that device.' So I started a program under the table with my fellow scientists. I knew that this project really couldn't succeed if you didn't resolve this technical hurdle."

Eventually, the first of several management changes occurred, and a new team took charge at CytoTherapeutics. The team put Tao in charge of the research effort, and she and her colleagues began to make significant progress. Most important, after much trial and error with various animal and human cells, Tao's team discovered a human cell line that could live inside a small, permeable capsule. It was a strain of human retinal cells, known as ARPE-19, which had been extracted from the eye of a 19-year-old man who died in a car accident in the 1980s. The line had been created by a biochemist at the University of California, Davis, Larry Hjelmeland, who himself was legally blind. It was one of many cell lines Tao's team had purchased from a national cell bank and tested.

As Tao and her colleagues were discovering the viable cell line, biomedical engineers John Mills and Konrad Kauper were refining the capsule invented by Aebischer. Mills and Kauper eventually came up with a polymer capsule, with walls as thin as a human hair. Inside was a tangle of tiny fibers, known as the scaffold, on which the cells grew. The capsule's pores were microscopic, small enough to keep out white blood cells and antibodies of the immune system, but large enough to let the therapeutic protein escape and oxygen and glucose enter.

"There was a bewildering array of variables involved in making the membrane, and when you add a biological component, it becomes almost like a black art," said Mills.

Tao and her colleagues had successfully made a capsule that contained viable retinal cells, but what was its potential therapeutic value? That became clear in 1998 when Tao met with Alan Laties, a well-known ophthalmologist from the University of Pennsylvania and chairman of the Scientific Advisory Board of the Foundation Fighting Blindness.

"He said, 'There is a disease particularly well suited for your device,'" recalled Tao. "'It's retinitis pigmentosa, a genetically linked degenerative disease for which there is no treatment. If you can show your technology will work for this, I'll support you all the way.'"

This was the beginning of a collaboration between Tao and Laties. Searching the scientific literature, Tao read about researchers who had successfully produced CNTF in cells. Using a genetic engineering technique, Tao's team manipulated the human retinal cells to make CNTF, a protein the retinal cells don't usually produce. They then placed the cells in the capsule, inserted the capsule into samples of fluid that mimicked conditions inside the eye, and found that the cells continued to thrive and crank out CNTF. They had succeeded in producing what one of them called a "micromachine."

"We needed cells to be able to multiply and live in a device for a long time," recalled Tao. "We needed cells to perform in highly unnatural conditions because in a capsule they have no access to blood supply. We wanted the cells to be strong and proliferate. And we had accomplished all that. We had basically unlocked the amazing potential of these cells."

As these breakthroughs were occurring, CytoTherapeutics acquired a California company, Stem Cell, Inc. Tao soon sensed a lack of enthusiasm for her ECT research and picked up hints that the Rhode Island operation might be closed. Nevertheless, Tao's team pressed on, working with University of Pennsylvania researchers to implant CNTF into the eyes of rats with retinitis pigmentosa. These experiments showed that the protein did indeed prevent photoreceptors from degenerating. The team then devised an experiment to implant a device with CNTF-producing cells into two Irish setters with retinitis pigmentosa. One would be a control animal, with no CNTF-producing cells. The other would receive the device with the therapeutic technology. Working with Cornell University, the researchers implanted the capsules and launched a seven-week study. Two weeks into the trial, however, in the summer of 1999, disaster struck.

CytoTherapeutics announced that it was shutting down the Rhode Island office and, with it, Tao's work. The management said that Tao and her colleagues had to leave that day and posted a security guard outside the building to search employees as they headed home. Frantic, Tao called Laties at the University of Pennsylvania and explained the situation. He asked for the name of CytoTherapeutic's CEO and said he would telephone him. Ten minutes later, Laties called Tao back, saying he had spoken with the CEO and explained the importance of her work to retinitis pigmentosa patients around the world. The CEO gave Tao and her team permission to remove their cell lines, notes, and other items related to their research.

The group carted boxes of material out of CytoTherapeutic's headquarters near Providence. Tao took reams of documents to her house. Several engineers carted away material to their basements and garages. A molecular biologist gave the cell samples to his wife, who worked at a Providence hospital and stored them there.

Several weeks later, the results of the Irish setter studies came in. Tao's colleagues took samples of retinal tissue and sent them to outside scientists for evaluation. The control dog had only two to three layers of photoreceptors in its retina. But the dog with the encapsulated cell technology had grown five to six layers of photoreceptor cells in seven weeks, a dramatic improvement and a strong sign that the technology might halt the progression of retinitis pigmentosa.

The team's elation over the results was tempered by the reality that they were professionally homeless. Working without pay for six months, Tao searched for a company that might acquire the rights to CytoTherapeutic's encapsulated cell technology and continue to fund research. She found what she was looking for in a small French biotech firm, Neurotech, which acquired the ECT rights and launched Neurotech USA in January 2000. At the time of its demise, CytoTherapeutics had consumed $120 million in start-up capital.

Infusing the venture with an additional $25 million from 2000 to 2005, Neurotech supported continuing research into using ECT. In 2000 and 2001, Tao's team performed experiments with forty more dogs with retinitis pigmentosa, and all showed an appreciable increase in photoreceptor cells after the treatment. Studies with rats, rabbits, and other animals showed similar results. Indeed, a device placed in a rabbit's eye was still producing CNTF eighteen months after implantation.

Meanwhile, studies of the disease in animals and humans showed that it was caused by more than one hundred genetic mutations that impair the metabolism of retinal cells.

"This all leads to the point where the cells do not sustain themselves and the end result is cell death," said Tao. "CNTF can enhance the activity of the cells and prevent them from dying."

The eye, it turned out, was the perfect place to insert an ECT device, as the body's immune system, for a variety of evolutionary reasons, is not as active there as in other parts of the body. And because of physiological barriers between the blood supply and the eye, degenerative retinal diseases weren't amenable to drug therapies. Many things came together to contribute to the success of Tao and her colleagues, including a bit of luck.

"What did Pasteur say? 'Chance favors the prepared mind,'" said Stabila, Neurotech's molecular biologist. "Every time we came to a crossroads, we had to make a decision. And it had to be the right decision, or otherwise you would have gotten lost in this maze. But we were very fortunate. Weng has always made the right decision. She's very insightful. She can see things others can't. You know those paintings that have a hidden image and you have to stare at them a long time before you really see what's there? That's what Weng can do."

By 2003, Neurotech was ready to test the safety of its device in humans. Persuading the federal government to approve the trials was not easy. Neurotech's work represented one of the first times an ECT capsule was being placed in a human. Company vice president William Tente, who oversees the manufacturing and regulatory side of the business, recounted the initial reaction to Neurotech's proposal.

"The perception of the regulators was, 'Oh, my God! You're going to put something in somebody's eye and you're going to put cells that are genetically engineered in the device in that eye?'" recounted Tente. "It was very tough."

Ultimately, after submitting a 4,000-page application, Neurotech won approval from the FDA and the National Eye Institute to proceed. The company was running into regulatory hurdles that never existed for early biomedical engineering pioneers, such as Earl Bakken. But this combination of cells, genetic engineering, and a new delivery system was taking biomedical engineering in a new direction, holding out the promise of a cure that traditional biomedical engineering was never able to achieve.

The news that a limited trial of ten patients would begin in October 2003 was greeted with joy at Neurotech. None doubted that without Tao it would not have come to pass.

"I call her the pit bull," said Stabila. "She's the toughest person I ever met. I have seen over the last eight years how she has been chewed out by so many people. But she knew that what we were doing was right, and that's why we've gotten where we are today. She is the only reason I stayed. Weng has built a culture here. We love what we do and believe in what we do. This may never happen again in these people's lives. We'd jump in front of a train for this project."

Cell biologist Brenda Dean added, "When it looked like we were closing down, I just felt that walking away would be like wasting eight years of my life. A lot of naysayers said this is never going to work. But Weng kept the group together, and we hung on. It's a great opportunity to see a therapy actually go into a human. Some people spend their whole careers in science and never get a chance to do that."

The FDA and National Eye Institute were concerned enough about testing the new device that they implanted it in a rolling fashion, inserting it in the first patient in October 2003 and in the tenth, and last, in November 2004. Five of the patients had advanced retinitis pigmentosa and could see very little. They were given low doses of CNTF. Five, including Dr. Theodore Hersh of Atlanta, had less severe cases and, though legally blind, still had varying amounts of vision. They were given higher doses of the regenerative protein. The devices were to stay in the patients six months, and the main goal was to make sure the devices were safe. The effectiveness of the encapsulated cell technology was not the primary concern of the regulators, although it certainly was to the patients, the youngest of whom was 32 and the oldest—Hersh—was 71.

Tao and Pam Heatherton—Neurotech's animal surgeon and the person who implanted ECT devices in the company's animal studies—recall the moment when they saw the first patient at the National Eye Institute in Bethesda, Maryland. She was accompanied by her husband and a Seeing Eye dog, a sight that brought home the reality that, after a decade of struggle, their device was about to be tested in a person who badly needed it.

"I welled up with tears," recalled Heatherton. "And for all the animals I sacrificed I said, 'Thank you. Thank you so much.'"

The procedure was simple. The surgeon anesthetized the eye and then inserted the tiny capsule into the upper temporal corner of the eyeball, where it remained out of the field of vision of the patients, who were conscious but sedated. The human retinal cells in the capsule then began secreting the CNTF into the vitreous humor and to the damaged photoreceptor cells of the retina, at the back of the eye.

A surgeon implanted the capsule in Hersh's right eye, the one most affected by retinitis pigmentosa, on June 9, 2004. Within a month Hersh began to notice changes in that eye. He showed "significant improvement" in reading the letters on a reading chart. He could see the faces of people on television more clearly and could distinguish colors better, as he learned during the coverage of the 2004 presidential election, when he could tell the difference between the red and blue states on the map. He could also read large captions on the television, which he couldn't before. And he noticed that when he closed his relatively good eye, he could see his face in the mirror when he shaved. Before the ECT, if he closed his good eye, he couldn't see well enough to shave.

"There are definite improvements with the capsule," Hersh told me. "I can see what's on the cover of *Time* magazine from 5 feet away and couldn't before. And I can get around a little better by myself."

Hersh is encouraged by the results and would like to have the device implanted in both eyes.

"I think they have a real contraption there," said Hersh, who, four months after the device was removed, still retained his improved vision. "If it's going to help me, imagine what it could do for a younger person, where the disease hasn't progressed as much. They wouldn't have to quit their profession. Imagine if I had had this earlier. I would still be teaching. I think this is a significant advance in stopping the progression of the disease. I don't want to use the word *cure.* It's not a cure. But for thirty years there's been nothing around that offered a glimmer of hope. This does. It's incredible."

Of the five patients who still retained a sizable percentage of their sight, three—including Hersh—reported marked improvement. Of the five with extremely advanced retinitis pigmentosa, however, only one showed improvement, a result, Tao believes, of the severe degeneration of their photoreceptor cells. Tao and her colleagues are guardedly optimistic that ECT therapy may indeed slow or halt the progression of retinitis pigmentosa in people with mild to moderate forms of the disease.

Neurotech will conduct wider trials of retinitis pigmentosa patients. And in the summer of 2005, the company is planning a trial with twenty-four patients who have another ailment, age-related macular degeneration. Affecting 13 million people, age-related macular degeneration is also a retinal disease in which photoreceptor cells are destroyed, which may make it suitable for treatment with encapsulated cell technology. Age-related macular degeneration, which wipes out the central field of vision, is the leading cause of vision loss among Americans older than 60.

Tao is aware that the promise of drugs and devices often fades in later-stage clinical trials, as large numbers of patients participate. But she is confident that Neurotech's therapy—with a proven track record in dozens of animal experiments—will stand up to further scrutiny. Indeed, she believes ECT for people with retinitis pigmentosa could win FDA approval and be on the market by 2010.

If that comes to pass, Tao's vision and resolve will have played a pivotal role in bringing a new biomedical technology to fruition. She overcame the opposition of numerous management teams, surmounted a host of scientific obstacles, and fought, at numerous junctures, to keep the ECT project from collapsing. Now, however, the indifferent CEOs are gone, and many of the technical challenges have been overcome. And Tao, her colleagues, and their new device show no sign of fading away.

"I know we've made a difference," said Tao. "We took something no one else thought was possible to achieve and we have done it. From the beginning I went into medicine to help people. And today we have patients who need help and had no hope, and now they have hope. For me, that is very satisfying."

CHAPTER 15

Tissues

By the spring of 2004, life with diabetes had become nearly intolerable for Laura Cochran. Her four young children were a handful, but motherhood would have been the usual manageable, rewarding chaos were it not for the illness that had attacked her body seventeen years before. At age 28, Cochran was stricken with Type 1 diabetes, the most serious form of the illness and one in which her body's own immune system attacked her pancreas, preventing it from making the insulin that converts sugar into energy for her cells. In May 2004, Cochran, from Columbus, Georgia, was among the 1.3 million Americans with Type 1 diabetes. That number paled in comparison with the 18 million Americans who had contracted Type 2 diabetes, many as a result of an epidemic of obesity sweeping the country.

If people with Type 1 are the sickest of all diabetics, then Cochran was among the sickest of the sick. In the parlance of the medical world, she was a "brittle" diabetic, meaning her blood sugar levels fluctuated wildly and often. And even though she was a model patient and equipped with state-of-the-art, diabetes-busting technology—including a small pump that administered the proper dose of insulin—she still was firmly in the grasp of the disease. Once, while nine months pregnant and driving her 7- and 10-year-old boys in the family van, she had a hypoglycemic attack and drifted in and out of consciousness. Only the shouted warnings of her sons kept her from running off the road.

"If someone had been walking on the side of the road or on a bike,

I would have killed them," recalled Cochran, a slender, stylish woman with shoulder-length brown hair. "You become very irrational, and I did not realize what was happening. . . . As a diabetic you bounce back and forth and at the end of the day you feel like a wrung-out dishrag. I could go from being in a perfectly stable mood to being an absolute bear, and my children bore the brunt of it."

In addition to living with such short-term effects, Cochran also had to confront the reality that because she had Type 1 diabetes her time on earth would likely be shortened by fifteen years. People such as Cochran are prime candidates for kidney failure, heart disease, vision loss, and neuropathy, the last of which occurs when tissue in the extremities dies from poor circulation.

"When I first got diabetes, they said there'd be a cure in five years," said Cochran, who worked as a sales representative for a corporate merchandise and logo company before retiring at age 40 to be a stay-at-home mother. "But you lose hope and you think, 'Do I have to live with this for the rest of my life?' When you're a diabetic you always fantasize about what you'll be doing when a cure comes. You dream of walking through the den and Peter Jennings is on TV announcing a cure and then you rush to the doctor and there will be a cure for you and millions of other diabetics."

In May 2004, Laura Cochran was not the recipient of a complete cure, but she experienced something nearly as good. And the way doctors finally helped her break the bonds of diabetes offers a glimpse into where medicine and engineering are heading in the coming decades as they try to regenerate, or create anew, ailing parts of the body.

At Emory University Hospital in Atlanta, surgeon Christian P. Larsen, director of the Emory Transplant Center, performed an operation on Cochran known as the Edmonton protocol. Named for the Canadian city where the procedure was first carried out by transplant surgeon James Shapiro and his colleagues, the Edmonton protocol involved the transplantation not of an organ but of cells. Using a pancreas from a deceased organ donor, Larson's team, employing a surprising combination of high- and low-tech methods, pulverized the pancreas and extracted 373,000 of that organ's signature rounded clusters of cells, known as islets. The islets produce the insulin that, in effect, directs the body's cells to take up glucose.

After gathering a slug of islet cells from the donor pancreas, Larson then injected them through a vein and into Cochran's liver. There, the pancreatic cells took up residence and, quite remarkably, began functioning as a miniature pancreas. Cochran's blood sugar levels stabilized, though she still needed some insulin, and two weeks later Larsen extracted 664,000 additional islet cells from a second donor pancreas and injected those into Cochran's liver. Since that day, Cochran no longer has diabetes. She has jettisoned the insulin pump and takes drugs only to prevent her body from rejecting the alien cells. Cochran was the 6th Georgian and roughly the 300th person worldwide to undergo the Edmonton protocol.

"It is miraculous," she told me on a scorching July day after visiting Emory for a two-month postoperative checkup. "When you get out of diabetes management, you realize how truly bad you felt. When you have diabetes, you get in that mind-set, and it becomes normal. And then to be able to come out of that and go a whole day without crashing and burning is a miracle. What amazes me is my energy level. I don't have to eat to keep up my glucose levels. I don't have to wear an insulin pump. I don't have to think like a pancreas. I just feel great. It just gives you so much freedom. I feel blessed that I was chosen to be in this study."

Cochran's happy ending, however, is far from typical. There is a severe shortage of donor organs in America and around the world, with 95,000 critically ill people in the United States alone on waiting lists to receive pancreases, hearts, livers, kidneys, and other organs. (In 2005, 4,100 patients were waiting for pancreases, 65,000 for kidneys, 18,000 for livers, 3,200 for hearts, and 3,900 for lungs. Waiting time for some organs can stretch three years, and many patients die before receiving an organ.) These figures do not include the millions in need of new blood vessels, cartilage, or other tissue transplants.

Biomedical engineers are working on a solution to the problem, although the challenges are immense. In Atlanta alone, researchers at the Georgia Institute of Technology, collaborating with their crosstown colleagues at the Emory University School of Medicine, are taking the initial steps toward figuring out how to create artificial pancreases, grow blood vessels in a laboratory, and coax severed nerves into reestablishing long-cut connections.

Investigators at scores of universities across the country are, with funding from the National Institutes of Health and the National Science Foundation, undertaking similar research projects, all with the audacious goal of making or regenerating parts of the body. This emerging field is known as tissue engineering, but a broader term, encompassing treatments like the Edmonton protocol, might be regenerative medicine. It is among the most promising, and most hyped, of all the spheres of biomedical engineering.

"There is a transplantation crisis in this country, and tissue engineering has the potential of confronting that crisis," said Robert M. Nerem, the director of the Georgia Tech / Emory Center for the Engineering of Living Tissues (GTEC). "There is a big discrepancy between the number of people needing organs and donor availability. The only way to provide that organ stream is by tissue engineering."

Michael Lysaght, director of Brown University's Center for Biomedical Engineering, put it this way: "For any terminal, end-stage organ disease you're much better off with a transplant. But getting an organ transplant is like landing on Boardwalk—great when it happens, but nothing you can depend on."

Although researchers dream of one day growing entire human organs, biomedical engineers are now tackling a more realistic goal: creating parts of an organ or inventing devices that contain human cells to take over an organ's function. Numerous researchers at GTEC are investigating ways, for example, to make heart valves, cardiac tissue, or blood vessels out of human cells. Another major area of research, both at GTEC and across the nation, is the creation of a capsule, perhaps no bigger than a computer chip, containing cells that would assume the functions of the pancreas in diabetics.

Tissue engineers also are researching methods of creating cartilage and bone in the laboratory. Already, one company, Genzyme Biosurgery, has developed a technique in which a pea-sized chunk of a patient's knee cartilage is removed and cultured in a lab to reproduce a larger piece of cartilage containing millions of cells. A surgeon then implants those new, tissue-engineered cells to heal a defect in a patient's knee. Roughly 2,000 patients a year are receiving implants with this technology, known as Carticel, but the market has not proved as large as Genzyme had hoped, in part because the tissue-engineered product does not work well in all patients. Many orthopedic surgeons still place more faith in time-tested joint replacement surgeries, performing 175,000 hip replacements and 365,000 knee replacements a year, numbers that dwarf those for Carticel therapy.

The halting success of tissue-engineering companies demonstrates the scientific and commercial challenges facing the field. Many leaders in tissue engineering warn against overselling the technology and raising patients' hopes. Even something as seemingly simple as a human blood vessel turns out to be devilishly difficult to create in the lab. An artery is not just a pipe but rather a multitiered construct lined on the inside by a single layer of endothelial cells, which are supported by smooth muscle cells. A human blood vessel has to be tough—expanding and contracting a few billion times in a lifetime—yet it also has to be highly elastic. In addition, its inner surface should not be prone to causing blood clots.

As the young researchers in Nerem's lab can attest, it's not easy to cook up such a vessel. You need the right mix of proteins, such as collagen, for strength, and you need elastin for suppleness. Creating the inner layer of endothelial cells is especially difficult. The cells aren't just passive organisms but are strongly influenced by their physical environment, such as the flow of blood over them or the constant pulsing of the vessel.

This problem is at the heart of the challenges facing tissue engineers. As researchers are discovering, the body's cells don't exist in a vacuum but rather operate in a three-dimensional environment in which a host of stresses, forces, and flows determine how they will function. In keeping with the inevitable march of biomedical engineering down to the genetic level, it's also clear that these physical forces activate different genes that control the production of the proteins guiding physiological functions.

For these reasons, tissue engineers have a keen understanding of the marvelous complexity of the human body.

"One of the things you appreciate," said Nerem, "is that we're nowhere near as smart as the great creator."

In the late 1990s and early 2000s, some researchers seemed to lose that sense of awe, talking up tissue engineering as if scientists would soon be assembling humans at the lab bench. One researcher predicted that entire human hearts, made from living tissues, could be produced within a decade—a forecast that now looks too optimistic by many decades. As I set about writing this book, I accumulated stacks of articles about all spheres of biomedical engineering. The fattest, by far, was the folder on tissue engineering. Press speculation about the bionic man and the "Six Million Dollar" man filled innumerable columns in newspapers and magazines, yet researchers today are still laboring over Petri dishes, struggling to replicate the most basic physiological processes.

Lysaght, who has closely followed the progress of tissue engineering, said the field has been marked by two distinct periods. The first, in the 1990s, saw a euphoric leap forward with $400 million to $600 million a year in private venture capital being pumped into tissue-engineering companies worldwide. In Boston, several groups of tissue engineers garnered international publicity for some early work in the field. One of the most prominent was Robert Langer, a biochemical engineer at the Massachusetts Institute of Technology who in the 1980s pioneered methods of controlled-released drug delivery by placing drugs and chemotherapy agents in degradable polymers. Anthony Atala, then of Children's Hospital in Boston and the Harvard Medical School, created artificial bladders, implanting them successfully in dogs and even several humans. Two brothers, Charles A. Vacanti and Joseph P. Vacanti—both now at Harvard University—rebuilt a portion of a patient's thumb using an artificial scaffold and the patient's own bone cells grown in the lab. German researchers grew a jawbone in a man's back and implanted it in his jaw. Progress was being made in developing artificial skin and cartilage. By 2001, 3,300 people were working in seventy tissue-engineering start-up companies worldwide, with a total investment of $3.5 billion, according to Lysaght.

Sales of tissue-engineering implants, however, never topped $40 million a year. And by 2002 the tissue-engineering bubble, like the Internet bubble of the late 1990s, had burst. Perhaps the greatest problem was the sheer complexity of re-creating organs and body parts. Even though some researchers managed what Lysaght calls "one-off" achievements, these were a far cry from the rigorous clinical trials needed to secure approval from the Food and Drug Administration. Indeed, the FDA's insistence that many tissue-engineering implants meet the same standards as drugs and biological products has been a major hurdle. Lysaght estimates that to bring a viable tissue-engineering product to market costs at least $100 million and takes at least a decade.

"Tissue engineering is Tomorrow-land," said Lysaght. "Tissue engineering was great initial science, was fast out of the blocks, then stumbled terribly with the first commercialization. The vision of tissue engineering is impeccable. But companies outran their logistical supply lines."

Lysaght and many others point out that some of the most important advances in biomedical engineering of the past sixty years, such as the kidney dialysis machine and the heart-lung bypass machine, were invented by surgeons or engineers with wide latitude to experiment on patients, some of whom died. Such freewheeling invention is far more difficult in today's rigorous regulatory climate.

Another problem facing tissue engineers is that although researchers may have succeeded in cobbling together a thumb or a jaw, the fundamental science behind these achievements is still not well understood.

"Development began to outrun research, and a lot of academics began to say, 'Let's get back to the basics,'" said Lysaght.

Even when tissue engineers have succeeded in creating an organ in the laboratory, as was the case with artificial skin, attempts to bring the product to market often have failed because it was too costly or there was minimal demand. One example is Advanced Tissue Sciences (ATS), which was based in San Diego. Founded in 1987, ATS raised and spent $350 million to develop a number of products, including two FDA-approved artificial skin materials known as Trans-Cyte and Dermagraft. Although the products were successful in replacing burned skin and treating pressure sores and skin ulcers, these treatments proved more expensive than existing therapies such as skin grafts or covering wounds with traditional dressings. After years of research and marketing, Advanced Tissue Sciences filed for bankruptcy in 2002. A successor firm, Smith and Nephew, now produces TransCyte and Dermagraft in limited quantities.

Gail Naughton, a tissue engineer and the former president and chief operating officer of ATS, said the company made two fundamental mistakes: tackling a problem—skin repair—for which alternative treatments already existed, and overestimating the size of the potential market.

"The biggest lesson I learned is that you have to go after something that has no cure, like Parkinson's or diabetes," said Naughton, now the dean of the College of Business Administration at San Diego State University. "If there is an acceptable treatment on the market, your battle is far greater."

Naughton also said that Advanced Tissue Sciences and other tissue-engineering companies that went bankrupt were badly hurt by an inordinately slow FDA approval process. The FDA took four years to approve the company's tissue-engineered skin for burns and seven years to approve its product for diabetic ulcers, delays that played a role in Naughton's company burning through its capital.

"None of the early biomedical engineering products, like pacemakers and heart valves, would be on the market if they had to go through the same trial process that we have to go through today," said Naughton. "These devices got into patients with no regulatory hurdles. Tissue engineering has had every hurdle thrown at it. Sometimes the burden placed on a new technology before it can start helping people is just onerous. There has to be some kind of balance."

Despite the sobering lessons of Advanced Tissue Sciences, Naughton is optimistic about the future of tissue engineering. She is a consultant to a company that, building on ATS's diabetic ulcer work, has invented a product that stimulates blood vessel growth in tissue. The company is investigating ways to use the product to encourage vessel growth in damaged heart muscle. Working with the tissue-engineered heart products, she said, is a sound business prospect because cardiologists and cardiac surgeons have a long history of embracing innovative technologies, such as pacemakers and defibrillators.

"I think tissue engineering will play a huge role," said Naughton, who also does consulting for a company researching therapies for Parkinson's disease. "A cure for diseases like Parkinson's or diabetes is what will turn around the field of tissue engineering."

Lysaght said the field is regrouping after the setbacks of recent years but will eventually play an important role in medicine.

"Where tissue engineering is headed now is not clear," said Lysaght, noting that the federal government is pouring large sums of money into tissue-engineering research. "The field has kind of lost its way. . . . But that doesn't invalidate the underlying science or the broad-scale vision. Look at the space race. In 1957 rockets were blowing up all the time. In 1969 we landed on the moon. A proper approach to past and present achievements is wonder. But the way to approach the future is with a dose of skepticism. You don't want to suspend your critical judgment."

One person who has maintained a skeptical view of the field is Martin Yarmush, chairman of the Biomedical Engineering Department at Rutgers University.

"I would say 50 percent of the so-called discoveries produced by tissue engineering are hype and salesmanship and flat-out nonsense," Yarmush told me. "A scientist tries to solve problems; not create buzzwords. . . . I call it science entertainment. . . . What has happened since the 1970s in many fields is the industrialization of scientific research, and industry needs to sell. So everything is always the best thing since sliced bread. Science used to be a noble art form, but now it's a business, and when it's a business, you don't finish the painting. You put together a little flour and a little water and you say, 'I've got a cake.' . . . There is a lot of good fundamental tissue-engineering work that will eventually make all the difference. But the problem is that there's so much hype that it trivializes the other work."

Yarmush also noted that while rudimentary lab research on tissue engineering is taking place, such work may become moot as industry researchers move rapidly ahead with alternative solutions to medical problems. One example, he said, is arterial stents coated with anticoagulants and other substances, which could reduce the need for tissue-engineered blood vessels. The continuing improvement of mechanical devices, such as left ventricular assist devices, may also reduce the need to create a tissue-engineered heart.

"Industry is selling thousands and thousands of stents," said Yarmush. "If you're married to a problem, you will eventually find a solution. But if you're married to a solution, you're dead if it's not a good one."

Nerem is more sanguine about the future of tissue engineering.

"There is no question that tissue engineering has been overhyped," he said. "But having said that, we now have twenty industrial partners. Nine years ago when some joined, they simply said we'll watch what's happening. All those companies are now doing some tissue engineering. The reality out there is that industry will lead to the next generation of medical implants, but it will not happen overnight. The industry is very much a fledgling industry. Some companies have gone belly-up, but some of the bigger ones are investing more and more. For tissue engineering to be successful it has to enter markets where there are not alternatives. The niche for tissue engineering has to be where you are doing something that no one else can do."

Tissue engineers today realize that the best chance for success lies in using the body to nurture or guide an implant, rather than inserting an alien device inside a patient. Prime examples of this would be a gel to stimulate the growth of severed nerve fibers, or an artificial scaffold on which a patient's bone or cells would be encouraged to grow. Another instance might be a patch of living cells that would replace damaged cardiac muscle and would integrate seamlessly into a patient's heart.

"In the next twenty years regenerative medicine is it," said David Archer, an Emory University neuroscientist collaborating with Georgia Tech biomedical engineers on ways to restore function to injured portions of the brain. "In a way it comes down to the body does it best. How can we take cells and reeducate them and put them in the right environment and have them do what we want them to do?"

In the biomedical engineering laboratories of Georgia Tech and Emory, back to basics is the order of the day. Indeed, what struck me most, after reading about some of the more sensational achievements of tissue engineering, was how fundamental the research is at places like Georgia Tech and Emory, which are a microcosm of tissue-engineering centers worldwide. Professors and graduate students there are trying to understand the building blocks of cells, bones, and organs. A few years of such labor gives those involved a profound respect for the cosmic handiwork of evolution. As Yarmush points out, you don't really appreciate the stunning efficiency of a pancreas or a liver until you try to make one yourself.

On a July morning in 2004, I visited graduate student Ann Ensley, who was making a blood vessel from scratch and then testing it to see how it might compare with the real thing. A researcher in Nerem's tissue-engineering lab, Ensley—an outgoing woman with thick, light-brown hair falling to her shoulders—first took a pig's carotid artery and, after exposing it to a series of chemical and heat treatments, extracted pure elastin. To this she added a healthy measure of smooth muscle cells from a baboon, which she obtained by culturing cells from a baboon artery. She threw in some collagen for strength and then, by altering the pH of this concoction and bringing it up to body temperature, produced a gel. She then molded the mixture in a test tube and wound up with an off-white, elastic vessel that resembled an artery or a vein.

What most interested Ensley was not the shell of the vessel itself but what would line the inside of it. Making a resilient vessel is critical, but equally important is creating a vessel that will not cause blood to clot, something that nature's own arteries accomplish when their inner lining releases substances that keep the blood speeding along. As she worked toward her Ph.D. in 2005, Ensley's goal was to create the single layer of cells lining the vessel, known as endothelial cells, and then subject them to the same forces and stresses they would encounter in the body to see how they reacted.

To make her own endothelial layer, Ensley extracted endothelial progenitor cells from a baboon's blood vessels. She then cultured those cells to create a large quantity, squirted those cells over a layer of collagen sitting in clear, plastic flasks, and bathed them in a pink-tinted growth medium. Ensley placed the flasks in a humidified incubator that would nurture the cells for three days at baboon body temperature, which is roughly the same as a human's.

After propagating millions of endothelial cells, Ensley extracted one of the flasks and showed me what the cells looked like. Placing a sample under the microscope, she pointed out how the cells had grown snugly against one another in the flask. They were a rounded, cobblestone shape, in contrast to the more elongated smooth muscle cells.

Seeking to mimic conditions in the body, Ensley placed eight slides with endothelial cells in another bioreactor and hooked them up to a series of pumps and tubes that shot a steady supply of liquid over the surface of the cells. As this flow, designed to roughly imitate circulating blood, bathed the cells, they slowly changed shape, elongating in the direction of the fluid flow. But what most interested Ensley was whether the simulation of blood flow would cause the cells to emit anticlotting substances, just as normal endothelial cells do.

To test this, she gently scraped off the endothelial cells from the 3-inch by 1-inch slides, collecting about 600,000 cells from each one. The cells formed a cloudy smudge in a mixture of formaldehyde, and she tested them with antibodies that would show their propensity to clot. In the end, Ensley's results were good: the endothelial cells inside a tissue-engineered vessel generally behaved like a normal vessel when exposed to blood flow, producing an anticlotting agent.

As part of her research, Ensley takes her tissue-engineered vessels to an animal lab in Oregon, where she sews them into an external shunt running from a baboon's femoral artery to its femoral vein. She then diverts the baboon's blood through the tissue-engineered vessel, which is lined with endothelial cells taken from the baboon's bloodstream. Her goal is not only to test the vessel's strength but also to see whether platelets in the baboon's bloodstream, which promote clotting, stick to the lining of the tissue-engineered vessel.

So far, the results have been mixed. She has succeeded in preventing platelets from sticking to the wall of the tissue-engineered vessel by creating sheer stress that matches the pressure in the baboon's artery. The news regarding the strength of the artificial vessel is less encouraging, as it tends to burst far more readily than real vessels. "The natural vessel is really strong and very similar to a rubber band—it's elastic and tough," said Ensley. "It's very hard to tear with your hands. I think of the tissue-engineered vessel as delicate. You can tear it with your hands."

Ensley is hardly disheartened by the results, seeing them as an integral part of exploring new bioengineering frontiers. Hers is the kind of spadework that tissue engineers are doing around the country. It is classic engineering and science—thorough, repetitive, full of dead ends. But this is the way science usually advances, not in great spurts but in plodding steps.

"I find it exciting," she said. "That's what research is all about. You've got to generate ideas. Many things could work. Many will not work. It's just a matter of trying them out until you find the one that does work. Research is really about learning, and each experiment teaches us something. On a day-to-day basis there will be failures, and you'll be really bummed. But the failures actually give us something that we use for the next experiment."

Like many biomedical engineers, Ensley—who is from a small town in North Carolina—was torn between a career in medicine and one in engineering. As an undergraduate at Georgia Tech, she majored in chemical engineering. The turning point for Ensley was when she went to work in the lab of Professor Ajit Yoganathan, a chemical engineer who has been doing biomedical engineering research for several decades. After helping Yoganathan and his graduate students with projects such as building heart models to determine the most efficient way to repair serious heart defects, Ensley was hooked. She realized she wanted to devote herself to bioengineering research.

"I got to understand what problems were being worked on and how I could really help contribute to the improvement of human health," recalled Ensley, who plans to work as a researcher at a biomedical engineering company after she gets her Ph.D. "When I looked at a career in medicine, there were few physicians out there doing innovative and cutting-edge work. I felt I could have more of an impact by being on the other side, by creating more devices and working with clinicians to bring new treatments to patients."

Ensley and Nerem collaborate with researchers from the lab of Dr. Elliot L. Chaikof, the chief of vascular surgery at the Emory University School of Medicine. A team of Chaikof's graduate students is looking for the right combination of elastin, collagen, and other substances to make a hardy artery or vein. Chaikof's group experiments with all manner of materials—including elastin that has been genetically engineered to be stronger—in the search for the ideal vessel material.

Chaikof may be a professor of vascular surgery, but he considers himself a "born-again, back-door bioengineer" intrigued by the possibilities of tissue engineering. An erudite man with curly black hair, he said surgery has advanced over the centuries from removal of diseased parts, to repair of the body, to reconstruction and replacement, and now to regeneration. A vital question his lab is tackling, said Chaikof, is "how do these biological building blocks that comprise tissues provide a useful starting point to develop a new class of materials or artificial organs and help in the repair or regeneration of the body?"

Chaikof said the need for tissue-engineered vessels, including those of smaller diameters, is "huge," whether it is for use in heart bypass operations, end-stage atherosclerosis, or revascularizing the legs of patients with multiple blockages in their lower extremities. Researchers at other universities are reporting some progress in encouraging tissue-engineered vessels to grow in animals. Rakesh Jain, a biomedical engineer at Harvard University, placed tissue-engineered vessels in a collagen gel and then implanted the gel mixture in mice. The vessels in the gel culture grew, formed branches, and began carrying blood.

In addition to making strong vessels, numerous labs, including Chaikof's, are investigating how to prevent clotting, a mechanism that exemplifies the complexity and exquisitely honed balance of human physiology.

"The body wants you to stop bleeding when you cut yourself, but when you're not bleeding, the body does not want the blood clotting," said Chaikof. "The challenge of having vessels of smaller size that can carry blood without clotting is daunting. But we want to see if we can emulate some of these processes and incorporate them into some of these materials. We're very interested in biologically inspired design. And we are slowly but surely making progress."

Chapter 16

Body Builders

At any given time, about 90,000 people are on the waiting list for new organs in the United States. Two-thirds of them are waiting for kidneys, while 15,000 to 20,000 desperately need a liver. A few thousand more wait, mainly in vain, for a heart. And then there are the hundreds of thousands of additional people, who, for various medical reasons, are not eligible for organ transplants. Many of them die, while others live on thanks to therapies such as kidney dialysis, which sustains about 300,000 people with end-stage renal disease in the United States.

These statistics, and the stories of patients such as Laura Cochran, testify to the overwhelming need to find a better way to treat people with malfunctioning organs. That challenge is one of the great goals of medicine and biomedical engineering today. Indeed, hundreds of researchers in academia and in the private sector are laboring to create cell-filled devices—some implanted in the body, some external—that will assume the functions of failing organs.

Given the epidemic proportions of diabetes in the United States, one of the most pressing research projects is the effort to invent a so-called bioartificial pancreas. At Georgia Tech, Professor Athanassios Sambanis, director of GTEC's Metabolic and Secretory Organ Program, is leading the university's investigations in this realm. Like other researchers, Sambanis—facing the reality that there is an acute shortage of donor pancreatic cells available for transplant—is exploring a number of avenues. One is to coax stem cells, the undifferentiated cells that eventually form various tissues and organs, to become like pancreatic islets. Another method is to see whether cells from the liver or the intestinal lining—which, like islet cells, react to the arrival of food and glucose—can, through genetic engineering, be turned into cells that would produce insulin. Sambanis, collaborating with colleagues at Emory, is working on ways to encapsulate clusters of insulin-producing cells that could be inserted in a person's abdominal cavity. The idea is that the polymer capsules would allow oxygen and glucose to get through, thus stimulating insulin production, while also simultaneously keeping out antibodies and the white blood cells seeking to launch an attack on the alien pancreatic cells.

Other biomedical engineers in the United States are looking at inorganic capsules that would resemble a computer chip, with insulin-producing cells on the inside and a superfine mesh regulating the flow of glucose and antibodies. This technique has enjoyed some success in mice but faces major challenges—including the inability to wall off all antibodies and the difficulty of keeping large numbers of encapsulated cells well nourished—before it will work in humans.

"Initially there's always enthusiasm, but the more we learn about these systems the more barriers we understand," said Sambanis, who earned his Ph.D. in chemical engineering but has gravitated to tissue engineering over the years.

Sambanis is intrigued with the possibility of manipulating cells known as "intestinal crypts." Found at the base of the villi—the tiny, fingerlike tendrils that line the intestine and aid in digestion—crypt cells make up 1 percent of the intestinal lining. An even smaller portion are crypt stem cells, which are of special interest to Sambanis and his colleagues. When a meal is consumed, these crypt cells secrete a hormone, called GLP1, that travels through the bloodstream to the pancreas and, in normal people, causes the secretion of insulin. Because of the close ties between the intestinal crypt cells and the pancreas, Sambanis believes they may be prime targets for genetic manipulation. They might then behave like pancreatic islets and release insulin in response to the rush of glucose that comes from food.

In late 2004, another company, Novocell of California, said it was close to conducting human trials using insulin-producing cells inside a patented polymer shell made of polyethylene glycol. The insulin-producing cells would be injected into the abdomen and would be replenished every twelve to eighteen months.

Sambanis predicted that it will be at least a decade before a bioartificial pancreas is ready for use in humans. "In ten years there will be major advances in cell-based research, but I'm a little bit doubtful that they will be in clinical use by then," said Sambanis. "We may be getting close. So the big improvement in quality of life for diabetics in the next five to ten years will be in the mechanical sphere. Beyond that the advances will be on the cellular and molecular level."

Meanwhile, a lucky few—the most severe diabetics—will be able to receive new islet cells through the Edmonton protocol. But even that procedure is not a sure bet for patients. Larsen has attempted to process enough islet cells from donor pancreases on seventeen occasions, nine of which produced enough high-quality cells for a transplant. And of those nine patients who received the protocol, five, including Laura Cochran, were able to stop taking insulin.

The dream of concocting an organ in a lab is alive and well at numerous other universities. One of the more promising efforts is under way at the University of Michigan Medical Center, where a team led by physician H. David Humes has invented what he calls a "bioartificial kidney." The device, already in human clinical trials, is designed to perform the functions of the kidney in patients with acute renal failure, which can be brought on by such conditions as a massive, systemwide infection, known as toxic shock, or loss of oxygen-rich blood due to massive bleeding. Acute kidney failure has a 50 percent mortality rate, yet 95 percent of people who experience such failure can eventually recover full kidney function if they survive the life-threatening episode.

Using Humes's technology, also known as a "renal kidney assist device," a patient's blood would be pulled out of his or her arm and run through two external cylinders. The first, employing existing technology, is a filter system designed to purify the blood of waste products. But the heart of Humes's device lies in the second cylinder, or cartridge, which contains about 7,000 hollow fibers seeded with roughly 1 billion human kidney cells cultured in a laboratory. Humes believes that the presence of the cells serves to counteract the flood of inflammatory molecules, or cytokines, that are present in the body during multiple organ failure.

In Phase 1 FDA trials, ten patients were treated with Humes's device. All showed significantly improved kidney function. Six of the ten survived more than thirty days, and the four who didn't survive perished from causes other than kidney failure. The first case involved a 29-year-old, 410-pound trucker who experienced multiple organ failure, including kidney failure, brought on by toxic shock. The patient was expected to die, but after being placed on Humes's artificial kidney, he resumed making urine and pulled through. Phase 2 FDA trials of 100 people were conducted in 2004 and 2005, and early results indicated that the kidney assist device was cutting patient mortality in half. Humes has created a company, Nephros Therapeutics, that has raised more than $50 million in private funding.

The company's goal is to develop an artificial kidney—ultimately implantable—to treat chronic or end-stage kidney disease. Those patients are now put on kidney dialysis and, on average, do not live more than five years from the beginning of dialysis treatments. Any implantable device will need to contain massive numbers of kidney cells on an extensive surface area of membranes, a challenge that will likely be met by new micromanufacturing techniques.

"There is an absolutely unmet medical need," Humes told a gathering of physicians and researchers at the Albert Einstein College of Medicine in New York City. "I want to address my talk mainly to the younger people here, as there is a world of opportunity to develop therapeutics for these unmet medical needs."

In 2005, Humes's device still faced numerous regulatory and technical hurdles; re-creating a human organ is a monumental scientific endeavor. To get a sense of how difficult it is to make an organ in a lab, you need look no farther than a project that Martin Yarmush of Rutgers, Professor Mehmet Toner at Harvard, and other collaborators are undertaking. They are attempting to develop an external artificial liver, or "liver assist device," a machine packed with liver cells that could sustain patients in acute liver failure. Yarmush is quick to point out the wondrously efficient design of the human liver, which contains 100 billion cells packed into a network of layers, lobes, and lobules. To duplicate that number of cells outside the body would require a surface more than 30 feet by 30 feet, which is obviously impractical. However, Yarmush and his collaborators are investigating the possibility of using only one-tenth that number of cells, packed into a relatively small external device, to help save the lives of people in acute liver failure. Researchers reason that the human liver, which is often self-regenerating, can still provide adequate function with only about 10 percent of its original mass. The largest organ in the human body, the liver serves many biochemical functions, including the detoxification of the blood.

An external artificial liver would be used to keep patients alive—including those who have been poisoned or have an acute illness—until their liver can regenerate or they can receive a transplant. Close to 2,000 Americans die each year from acute liver failure. Thousands more die waiting for transplants. Two companies have performed limited human trials with liver assist devices, although none has yet been approved by the FDA.

The greatest obstacle facing Yarmush's team is the source of liver cells, known as hepatocytes. Animal sources are plentiful, but human cells would be ideal. Researchers must arrange the hepatocytes in a relatively small device that will deliver blood or plasma to the cells without creating so much force, or sheer stress, that the cells will be damaged or killed. "You've got to keep the cells happy," said Yarmush, a large, bearded man with a wry sense of humor and a blunt manner.

Yarmush and his colleagues have done initial rat experiments in which they inject a toxin into the animals and then treat them with a small artificial liver device. In one comprehensive study, half of the rats survived, versus none in the control group. Yarmush also pioneered methods to keep liver cells alive and functioning well for weeks outside the body, a significant achievement.

But he is less sanguine about transferring such therapies to humans anytime soon.

"A home run in this field would be figuring out how to regenerate hepatocytes in the lab," said Yarmush. "If you could sprinkle magic dust on liver cells and have them grow, you'd have a competitive prototype device in five years."

The one area in which tissue engineering has begun to stick its foot in the clinical door, however tentatively, is in the realm of the body's hardware—skin, bones, and cartilage. The benefit to patients is potentially enormous. Roughly 21 million Americans have osteoarthritis, a degenerative disease that eats away cartilage, causing the painful rubbing of bone on bone. Tissue engineers are investigating methods of producing cartilage, a breakthrough that could eliminate the need for many of the more than 600,000 joint replacement surgeries performed each year in the United States. Tissue-engineered bone would have obvious uses in bone grafts.

As researchers gradually understand how the body's skeletal system is formed, with a mix of genetic signals and physical forces combining to produce joints and bone, the road map for tissue engineering is becoming clearer. At Georgia Tech and other research centers, tissue engineers are intent on creating substances and scaffolds that, once implanted in the body, will encourage cells to attach and help the body heal itself. This is where "regenerative medicine" and tissue engineering meet.

Barbara Boyan, the deputy director of the Georgia Tech/Emory Center for the Engineering of Living Tissues, is urging the young researchers under her charge to keep things simple and devise ways to let the body do the repair work. She has followed this strategy in inventing patented polymer scaffolds that can repair areas where bone and cartilage join. The scaffold, which dissolves after three months, enables cells in contact with bone to become bone cells and cells in contact with cartilage to become cartilage cells. A company she helped found, OsteoBiologics of San Antonio, also is marketing an FDA-approved bone graft substitute.

"We designed it so the body will heal itself," said Boyan. "In a lot of cases the body has tremendous regenerative powers. We're struggling too hard to make something outside the body. We need something that you put in the body and the body itself will help this differentiation occur. We need to understand the physiology of cells in the body and then design materials that mimic what's inside the body. . . . As we understand basic biology better, we can improve how we approach tissue engineering."

Her experience in the private sector has convinced her that many academics are too theoretical and need to have a more practical, market-oriented slant to their research.

"I've already worked with companies, and they're 15,000 steps closer to real practice," she said. "My original ideas were quite naive and not unlike the issues you find now in tissue engineering. When I have a conversation with tissue engineers, they want to make the products too complicated. You need to suit the user, and the user is not the patient. The user is the surgeon. You need to have a surgeon come in and say this is really what I need right now. For tissue-engineered products many people are trying for perfection. They're setting the bar too high."

Boyan's lab at Georgia Tech does much practical research but also conducts more long-range, theoretical investigations. On the practical side, graduate student Alice Zhao has been placing bone cells on different steel surfaces to see how the surfaces affect growth. She has found that bone cells grow particularly well on a surface that is both sand-blasted and acid-etched, something that might be useful in engineering future bone implants.

"Cells recognize the surface on which they live," said Boyan. "They get messages from the physical surface. . . . We try to understand what cells do if you give them signals more like conditions in real life."

In another Georgia Tech lab, associate professor Robert E. Guldberg is investigating several vital issues in orthopedic tissue engineering: how physical forces in the body shape the growth of bone and cells, how growth factors can be used to stimulate cartilage and bone growth, and how tissue-engineered scaffolds can be integrated into the body. A major problem with tissue-engineered bone is making it sufficiently strong.

"You get the M&M effect," said Guldberg, the director of GTEC's Orthopaedic Tissue Engineering Program. "It's strong on the outside and weak on the inside."

Guldberg is hopeful these problems can be overcome, and he is working on a polymer scaffold that would be used to help close bone gaps in people born with bone defects. Experimenting with mice, he has successfully seeded bone marrow cells onto the scaffold, although they have yet to completely fill in the scaffold and close the gap. He is applying a host of engineering skills, including computer modeling and imaging scaffolds with CT scans, to improve the structure and performance of the scaffolds. He also has attempted to make cartilage in the lab but, like other researchers, has had difficulty integrating the cartilage into the body so it can perform its function as a connective tissue.

In Guldberg's lab, graduate student Chris Gemmitti is studying ways to make cartilage, a bloodless tissue consisting of water and collagen. Cartilage, which Gemmitti likens to a stiff sponge, does not regenerate after it is torn or damaged, so the demand for a strong, easily implantable cartilage would likely be high. The challenge Gemmitti and others face is how to get cartilage to grow and attach to bone.

Carticel, the cartilage cell injection therapy by Genzyme, has worked well in some patients, says Gemmitti, but not enough to win over large numbers of surgeons. He is experimenting with ways not only to make cartilage with the right amount of the proper collagen, known as Type 2, but also to apply different physical forces that will strengthen it.

Gemmitti's passion about applying the rigors of engineering to the many unanswered questions in human physiology is typical of biomedical engineers.

"When I was young, I was one of those kids that loved taking stuff apart that wasn't broken, driving my father up a wall," said Gemmitti. "Biomedical engineering is really an underrated profession. Traditional engineers may look at biomedical engineers crossways, and say, 'You know a little about a lot and not a lot about a little.' But I think biomedical engineering is very, very creative. I love being an engineer and working on the greatest machine that has ever graced the earth—the human body."

One of the farthest frontiers of tissue engineering, and one that holds out potentially great rewards for millions of patients, involves the brain and the nervous system. On the scale of the possible, the most realistic objective is regrowing nerves of the peripheral nervous system, such as those in the hands and legs. And on the far end of that scale is the effort to restore damaged nerves in the central nervous system—the spinal cord—which to date has proven to be among the greatest challenges in medicine. Somewhere in between is repairing or replacing destroyed brain cells, such as inserting dopamine cells to treat people with Parkinson's disease.

One of the leaders of GTEC's efforts in neural tissue engineering is a 36-year-old biomedical engineer named Ravi Bellamkonda, a graduate of Brown University. He and his colleagues in the Biomedical Engineering Department are attacking several major problems, operating on the theory that they need to nudge the brain and nervous system in the right direction and then let it take over the work.

"It's not about just introducing an inert material into the body," said Bellamkonda. "The inert material strategy was not working. That shift in thinking gave rise to tissue engineering. We wanted to design cells to get a reaction, to be incorporated into the host, which inert materials do not do. We wanted cells to remodel because in our bodies everything is recycling and changing. The promise of tissue engineering is implants changing dynamically with time. The question is, can we evoke a positive reaction to promote healing?"

Bellamkonda and other investigators around the country have succeeded in coaxing peripheral nerves to grow 10 millimeters, or about four-tenths of an inch. But larger gaps between nerves have proved much harder to bridge. Researchers in Bellamkonda's lab are experimenting with laminin-1, a protein associated with nerve growth. They also are investigating the different physical or chemical cues that stimulate nerve growth. Nerves need an anchor on which to grow, and in the body they follow blood vessels or other tissue. Researchers are growing nerves on different surfaces—rough versus smooth, convex versus concave—to see which are the most salutary for nerve growth. Other scientists in Bellamkonda's lab are experimenting with different chemical cues to encourage nerve growth, with the tentacles following a stimulus much the way a human might follow the smell of baking cookies into the kitchen.

Should tissue engineers like Bellamkonda succeed in growing peripheral nerves, such a therapy would have many uses. Men who undergo surgery for prostate cancer, for example, often only get 40 to 50 percent recovery in severed nerves sewn back together by surgeons. The procedure leaves many men impotent, but a reliable way of bridging gaps in severed nerves could help solve that problem. Likewise, the success of conventional nerve graft surgery is about 25 to 40 percent, but an effective technique of tissue-engineered nerve growth would offer patients far better odds.

On the far tougher front of restoring connections in severed spinal cords, Bellamkonda's lab is pursuing several avenues of research. In spinal cord injuries, the greatest obstacle to restoring function is the scar tissue that forms around the traumatized area. Scar tissue blocks the transmission of nerve impulses, and Bellamkonda's group is probing ways to prevent the scar tissue from forming or methods to make the damaged cells immune from scarring.

"For me, from an engineering perspective, it's like a gold mine," said Bellamkonda. "The biologists say, 'The road looks like this. This is what is cut, and these may be important molecules affecting regeneration.' But they're not good at rebuilding that road by reconstructing pathways using those molecules, and that's where we come in. We are talking about biology, but we're talking in terms of design criteria—how to design new systems to get these things to work."

Around the country, researchers have reported mixed success with experiments in spinal cord regeneration. The Vacanti brothers, Charles and Joseph, of Harvard, reported in 2000 that they implanted immature neural cells in the severed spinal cord of a rat, enabling the animal to stand and walk after several months. Other researchers have been skeptical, saying that what the Vacantis saw as walking was little more than a reflexive response to the implant. Most tissue engineers believe that science is still years away from regenerating damaged spinal cords and enabling paraplegics or quadriplegics to walk on their own.

In brain tissue engineering, Bellamkonda and his research team are experimenting with different materials or scaffolds that would potentially enable transplanted stem cells or dopamine cells to survive in a person's brain. Tissue engineering will also undoubtedly play an important part in the burgeoning field of stem cell research, which may one day provide treatments for a host of neurodegenerative diseases, from Alzheimer's to multiple sclerosis.

No one, least of all Bellamkonda, expects a quick solution to any of these problems. But he is encouraged that across America hundreds of biomedical engineers and other scientists are doing fundamental research to seek cures for devastating conditions such as Alzheimer's and spinal cord injuries.

"Why would I travel 8,000 miles from India, when my parents are in India and my kids can't play with their cousins?" said Bellamkonda, a lean man with dark eyes and a thick head of black hair. "The reason is we have the best graduate and biomedical engineering programs in the world, and it allows us to work on problems and not see solutions for ten or twenty years. But we know we have to do this if we're going to solve these problems. I think I'm fortunate to work in a system where we have the privilege of figuring this out."

The great unknown, and the most alluring promise, of tissue engineering is stem cell therapy. Patient advocates—such as Michael J. Fox, who has Parkinson's, and the late Christopher Reeve—have placed high hopes in stem cells. Scientists now know that stem cells—the undifferentiated cells that can become any kind of tissue, from brain neurons to pancreatic islets—are found throughout the body. Embryonic stem cells are the progenitor cells that eventually differentiate into the roughly 200 cell types in the human body. But different kinds of stem cells exist in the bone marrow, blood, some organs, even body fat. The major challenge is to determine what combination of factors—genetic, chemical, physical, and mechanical—shapes cells and causes them to turn into tissue as different as the brain and the heart. Biomedical engineers are positioned to play a significant role in this effort, since they have the tools to analyze and model such a multifaceted process. But finding these cells and manipulating them to become certain kinds of tissue are two very different tasks, and progress has been arduous.

Still, the potential benefits are huge, particularly in the neurological area. The prospect of such a payoff is spurring governments, universities, and private companies worldwide to pour large sums of money into stem cell research.

In America, the driving factor today is the decision by California voters, in November 2004, to allocate $300 million a year to stem cell research for a decade. The successful referendum, supported by Governor Arnold Schwarzenegger and 59 percent of Californians who voted, will lead to a $3 billion investment in stem cell research. That sum dwarfs federal spending on stem cell studies, which in 2004 was $25 million and limited to a small, preexisting number of stem cell lines.

Other states, not wanting to be left behind in the twenty-first century's bioengineering revolution, are following suit, giving a huge impetus to stem cell research. Richard J. Codey, the acting governor of New Jersey, said his state would spend $380 million on stem cell research, calling it "the race for the cure." The governor of Wisconsin, Jim Doyle, said his state, spurred on by the California initiative, would spend $750 million on its biotechnology sector and on stem cell research. Like California governor Arnold Schwarzenegger, these governors understood that major investments in stem cell research would attract biotechnology firms and catalyze economic growth.

Major universities outside California also are gearing up to study stem cells, including Harvard, which is creating a $100 million stem cell institute. Overseas, scientists in Europe, China, Australia, New Zealand, and Japan all are plunging into stem cell work.

"The California stem cell initiative is the 800-pound gorilla," said Michael Lysaght of Brown University. "It will be the definitive event in tissue engineering and regenerative medicine in the next decade."

The field is attracting some of the brightest biomedical engineers. At Georgia Tech, Taby Ahsan, a postdoctoral student in Nerem's lab, is conducting experiments with embryonic stem cells from mice, as well as with human stem cells from bone marrow or fat. Her goal is to place these stem cells in a three-dimensional environment, apply a wide variety of forces, and see what role those forces play in turning the stem cells into different kinds of tissue.

"There's no roadmap to these experiments, there's nothing to tell me to do this or that," said Ahsan. "It's going to take a lot of different experiments, and it takes time. But that's the only way to start.

"We all quote these humanitarian reasons for why we're doing this work, but at the end of the day we just enjoy it. Being at the interface of biology and engineering is fun. And I really do think we'll have an impact on patients in my lifetime. It will be nice to say that we helped advance people's lives. . . . I see all these complexities and I am overwhelmed. I can't put the whole puzzle together, but maybe I can tell you how to make one piece of the puzzle. There are many ways to skin this cat."

Chapter 17

The Road Ahead

The future of biomedical engineering is on display at the University of California, San Diego, and it is invisible.

For more than half a century, the great achievements of biomedical engineering have been devices you could see and touch: heart pacemakers and defibrillators, artificial joints, ultrasound and CT scanners, implantable pumps to assist the heart, automated blood analyzers, kidney dialysis machines, cochlear implants, pulse oxymeters. But in the first decade of the twenty-first century, scientists in the vanguard of biomedical engineering are looking beyond these machines and instruments and setting their sights on the infinitesimal. Their goal? To bring the tools of engineering to bear on genetics and molecular biology and thereby cure now intractable diseases.

The genome may sound as if it belongs squarely in the domain of biologists, but biomedical engineers at UC San Diego (UCSD) contend that no group is better suited than engineers to make sense of the stunning complexity of genetics and the mountains of data it has produced. Nor, these researchers argue, is any discipline as qualified to tease apart the intricate relationships of 20,000 to 25,000 human genes and the roughly 30,000 proteins they produce, all of which make up human physiology and disease. Engineers are at their best when working with systems—mechanical, electrical, chemical, or biological—and in trying to understand the building blocks of life, the profession is taking on the most complicated system it has ever encountered.

"The more you dig, the more you find, and the deeper the hole gets," said Jeff M. Hasty, an assistant professor of biomedical engineering at UCSD whose lab is endeavoring to understand the network of genes that governs a simple organism like baker's yeast. "One of the first steps we're trying to figure out is which genes talk to which genes. Proteins also talk to each other and also talk to genes. How are they all connected? If I handed you a twenty-page circuit diagram of a VCR and said, 'Okay, go program it,' what would you do? You'd need a manual, and we need manuals to describe how these gene circuits work. But we're finding that the more you look at things you think you understand, the more they become coupled to other things, which are coupled to even more things."

Spend any time with scientists like Hasty and you quickly gain an appreciation for the nearly unfathomable intricacy of our genes. Each cell nucleus contains twenty-three chromosomes, made up of long strands of our genes. These tens of thousands of genes are composed of roughly 3 billion molecular building blocks of DNA. Such towering numbers can be crunched only by very powerful computers under the control of accomplished engineers and biologists.

As Michael Savageau, chairman of the Department of Biomedical Engineering at the University of California, Davis, put it, "For a long time biologists were so successful that they didn't need our help. But with the human genome project there was a recognition that there was a flood of data that was terribly important. Most biologists realized that they couldn't deal with all this data. They didn't have the computer skills. And engineers and mathematicians realized that, 'Hey, we can really make a contribution here.' All of a sudden there was a whole new way of looking at things. Biologists had been successful with a reductionist approach, but everyone began to understand that we've got to pull all this information together."

That is what biomedical engineers are doing at UCSD and at leading universities across the country, such as Berkeley, Stanford, Harvard, and the University of Washington. Efforts to plumb the mysteries of the genome and protein production go by a host of buzzwords, including systems biology, computational biology, bioinformatics, "in silico" biology—as in silicon chips and computers—proteomics, and even the unwieldy "interactomics." But no matter the catch phrase, all the jargon boils down to one thing: using massive computing power and the engineer's tools of mathematics and modeling to tackle one of the greatest challenges in the history of science.

"Biologists have tended to work on one thing at a time," said Shu Chien, the chairman of UCSD's Bioengineering Department. "But genes work as a circuit, as a whole. They are all linked together. In biology there was a lack of tools to bring everything together. To do that you need an engineering approach."

The payoff, when it comes, could revolutionize medicine and health care. Should biomedical engineers, biologists, and physicians succeed in unraveling how genes switch on and off, how they interact with one another, how they interact with proteins—simultaneously issuing commands for the proteins to be created and then, in turn, being affected by those same proteins—the clinical value would be enormous. Some researchers envision a day when a person gives a small sample of blood that is then used to rapidly sequence that person's genes, providing doctors with a map of how to treat illness with drugs or gene therapies targeted specifically at an individual's unique physiology. Some call this scenario the "personal genome" project.

"This will be the world of pharmacogenetics, where we determine your genotype, determine your propensity to get certain diseases, and determine your treatment," said Bernhard Palsson, a professor of bioengineering at UCSD and an expert in systems biology and genetic circuits. "That's what people hope will happen, that there will be tailor-made treatment on an individual basis. The idea is that you take people's blood once a year and it will be like getting your car tuned up."

Several companies already are marketing postage-stamp-size devices known as "genome on a chip," which contain samples of all known human genes. Labs can then place tissue from a cancer biopsy or a diseased liver on the chip, which indicates the genes being expressed by the tissue. This technology, also known as a DNA microarray, enables doctors and drug companies to rapidly screen for signs of pathological genetic expression or to test which drugs may be suppressing or activating genes.

In addition, numerous laboratories already have developed blood tests that can identify whether a person has a higher likelihood of being stricken with more than 1,000 diseases, including colon cancer and melanoma. Mirroring the growth of this emerging technology is the number of genetic counselors in American hospitals, which rose from 1,000 in 1993 to 2,300 in 2004.

Genetic screening is already being used to fashion treatment for individuals with certain types of cancer. In breast cancer, for example, about 25 percent of patients have tumors that overexpress a gene known as HER2—human epidermal growth factor receptor 2. This overexpression can cause rapid cancer growth and metastasis. But a genetic screening test can determine whether a patient overexpresses HER2, and the biotechnology firm Genentech has developed a drug, Herceptin, that targets the HER2 receptors on the outside of cancer cells. To date, Herceptin has shown some success in shrinking tumors and in increasing survival rates of breast cancer patients. It is just one of a group of molecular cancer therapies now coming onto the market and an early example of how genetic screening could lead to individualized treatment in the future.

Another weapon that may play a vital role in treating diseases—ranging from Parkinson's, to diabetes, to cancer—is the use of technologies so small that scientists had to coin a new prefix for it: "nano," which means one-billionth of something. Nanotechnology has been a much-hyped new field, but despite the hoopla, it shows promise. Using crystals that are 10,000 to 50,000 times thinner than a strand of human hair, nanotechnology has the potential to help image the body and then deliver therapies on a molecular and genetic scale. Biomedical engineers at UCSD are investigating the uses of nanoparticles and similarly minuscule "quantum dots." They also are researching ways to use somewhat larger devices—micro-electrical-mechanical systems (MEMS)—to create artificial pancreases and livers that could be implanted in patients.

To Taylor Sittler, a medical student at the University of Massachusetts, the lure of applying engineering to the human genome proved irresistible. After completing his second year of medical school, Sittler received a fellowship from the Howard Hughes Medical Institute to work on a master's degree in biomedical engineering with Trey Ideker, another of UCSD's "systems biology" wizards. For his thesis, Sittler is measuring the expression of various genes to try to predict the toxicity of different drugs on cultured liver cells. Should Sittler and others perfect ways to screen drugs on cultured human liver cells, it could radically accelerate and expand the process of drug testing, which would have great medical benefits.

After receiving his master's degree in 2005, Sittler planned to return to medical school. He may eventually do medical research, practice medicine, or both. In any case, he believes that in his lifetime the unraveling of the genome's mysteries will provide a wealth of information to doctors and patients, eventually making today's diagnoses look primitive.

"There will come a time when we're really going to be integrating much more information about biology than we can now," Sittler, 29, said while sitting in a lab near dishes of liver cells growing in incubators. "I'd really like to see us take more and more information into the clinic. I think that just as the Internet has brought the world to an individual's desktop computer, systems biology will bring much more information to the physician's Palm Pilot. You'll be able to make a much richer diagnosis without having to send the patient to five or six specialists. You will be able to do a genetic microarray [test] and the oncologist can look at it and the radiologist can look at it and there will be a whole level of integration of knowledge that we don't have now. In the end it will give much more power to the primary care physician."

The University of California, San Diego, is located less than a mile from the Pacific Ocean in the eucalyptus-covered hills of La Jolla. The Bioengineering Department, part of the Jacobs School of Engineering, is housed in a handsome, four-story building of pale stone and glass. Many of the department's labs are devoted to genetic research, and Trey Ideker's is typical: a quiet place where, often as not, Ph.D. and postdoctoral students sit in front of computers or small machines that can measure gene expression.

To probe how genes interact with other genes and proteins, Ideker has chosen to work with the simplest of all eukaryotic organisms. (Eukaryotes, which include humans, have one or more cells with distinct nuclei.) Ideker and his team have brought their considerable brainpower to bear on yeast, which may sound like a mismatch, until you realize that yeast has 6,000 genes, about a quarter as many as humans, and that many of them interact in ways that have yet to be understood. Forty percent of yeast genes are homologues, meaning they are similar to those of humans and other eukaryotic creatures, a fact that is of intense interest to Ideker and other researchers.

Why start with the yeast genome, rather than the human genome? "It's kind of like figuring out how an old television set works before figuring out how a new one works," said Ideker, a boyish-looking 32-year-old scientist with straw-colored hair.

The yeast genome, like its human counterpart, has been sequenced, meaning that scientists have unfurled the double-helixed DNA architecture of its nucleus and read out the four digital letters that, in long strands, contain the code for its replication and functions. (DNA is made up of long chains, or polymers, joined together by bridges known as nucleotides. The four nucleotides are A, C, G, and T, short for adenine, cytosine, guanine, and thymine.) Even though the yeast genome has been sequenced, that doesn't mean that investigators have a clear idea of what it all means. Indeed, as of early 2005, scientists didn't know the function of 40 percent of the 6,000 yeast genes, just as many human genes remain a mystery. Researchers liken sequencing the genome to having a list of all the words in the dictionary but not knowing the definition of many of them.

Ideker's goal is to match the words with definitions, to decode which genes—or combinations of genes—are responsible for which functions. To accomplish that task, Ideker, the son of University of Alabama biomedical engineer Ray Ideker, likes to engage in what he terms "reverse engineering." Forward engineering is when you build something, such as a plane, from scratch. Reverse engineering is when something, such as a yeast cell, already exists and you take it apart to see what makes it tick.

One way biomedical engineers do that is to perform experiments with regular yeast cells and compare them with yeast cells in which genes have been "knocked out," or removed. Already, researchers know that about 1,500 genes are essential to the life of the yeast cell, as became evident when researchers knocked out those genes and the cells died. Other genes might be crucial to the yeast cell's ability to grow or metabolize sugar, which also becomes clear when, one by one, genes are knocked out and compared with regular yeast cells. By screening regular yeast genes and knockout genes with antibodies, Ideker's lab can identify which genes are programmed to produce certain proteins. Through such tedious and time-consuming work, Ideker hopes to eventually construct an intricate diagram of all 6,000 yeast genes and the myriad proteins they create. This, in turn, may shed light on the function of thousands of human genes.

The ultimate goal, said Ideker, is to create a diagram of a yeast cell and all its gene/protein interactions, followed by similar diagrams of human cells. One benefit of such an accomplishment is that engineers and chemists could model the effects of drugs on cells.

"The reason we get out of bed in the morning is that once we have a cell diagram we can use that to test drugs on cells, long before human trials," said Ideker. "We could use computer simulations to figure out what drugs work against disease and which drugs have toxic side effects. If you're Boeing, you simulate plane design on your computers. Car manufacturers do the same thing. Why is it that the drug industry is one of the few modern industries that doesn't use computer simulation? The reason is that they did not build the cell, so we have to figure out how the cell is built."

When I visited Ideker's lab, his team of graduate students was performing experiments on a key area of interest: which genes and proteins are involved in repairing damage to DNA. The answer to this question is of great concern to the medical community, since DNA damage—from toxins, radiation, oxidation, or severe inflammation from diseases such as ulcerative colitis—can cause genetic mutations and cancer.

"We want to look at DNA damage and how the cell responds by turning on proteins," said Ideker. "Hundreds of proteins can be involved in recopying damaged DNA and repairing it."

In the lab, postdoctoral student Kai Tan was inducing DNA damage to yeast cells by exposing them to hydrogen peroxide. Then, working with lab manager Scott McCuine, Kai tested which of the 6,000 yeast genes were activated to repair the damaged DNA by ordering up proteins. Kai and McCuine used a microarray technology that involved placing all 6,000 yeast genes on a 1-inch by 3-inch chip that was fed into a machine the size of a large bread box. The machine then identified which genes had "turned on" to fix the peroxide-damaged DNA, labeling the activity of the genes by their color and brightness. That result was compared with a microarray scan of undamaged yeast.

In the lab of Bernhard Palsson, researchers also are studying lower-order organisms that have no nuclei, such as the *Escherichia coli*, or *E. coli*, bacteria, to understand how genes interact and affect cell metabolism. A native of Iceland, Palsson said the remarkable genetic similarity of so many species provides scientists with rich opportunities to study the human genome.

"The components you and I are made up of are incredibly similar to the components of a tree or bacteria," said Palsson, a youthful-looking man of 47 with a fondness for wearing blue jeans and baseball caps. "And it's the incredible way that it all comes together that makes up systems biology. Look, the *C. elegans* nematode [worm] has 18,000 or 19,000 genes. That's a slimy undignified organism living underground. But just add 7,000 genes and all of a sudden you have something that you have to send to college. It's all a question of how it comes together."

To explain the enormous complexity of his work, Palsson falls back on a relatively simple comparison between systems biology and a city's traffic flow. Sequencing the genome of yeast, *E. coli*, or a human being is akin to giving a motorist a map showing streets, some with names, some without. But to understand how traffic is flowing at any given time, a motorist needs to know when traffic peaks and ebbs, what roads merge and create bottlenecks, what drawbridges may be up or down at a given time, and where there is an accident. The street map lays out the bare bones structure, but only by grasping the intricacies of traffic rhythms and patterns can a motorist understand how the system works. The system's pathological state is a traffic jam, and in analyzing the factors that caused it—an accident or a flood of rush-hour traffic—a motorist can come to know the network and learn to circumvent its pathologies. The same holds true for systems biology, and biomedical engineers are trying to grasp the interplay of genes that leads to various diseases—and hence their treatments or cures.

Using the tools of systems biology, Palsson and his assistants have succeeded in developing a computer model that predicts which genetic mutations in red blood cells will cause chronic anemia and which will cause a milder form. Anemia is brought on by a deficiency of red blood cells or hemoglobin, and the red blood cell, which does not have a nucleus, is one of the simplest cell forms in the human body. By compiling the extensive research done on red blood cells and their genetics, Palsson's group was able to model which of 150 genes would cause the more severe form of anemia. Their model, completed in 2002, was one of the first uses of systems biology to predict disease based on the interactions of numerous genes and proteins.

Palsson's lab also has constructed a computer model of how 1,010 *E. coli* genes interact and control the organism's metabolism.

When I met Palsson in late 2004, systems biology was less than a decade old. And in those ten years—beginning with the sequencing of the first genome, a bacterium that causes meningitis and ear infections (*Haemophilus influenzae*), in 1995—biomedical engineers grappling with genetics had gone from a "data poor" to a "data rich" environment, Palsson said. Indeed, the graduate students in his lab were inundated with genetic data as, by early 2005, the genomes of close to one hundred organisms—everything from the dog to the malaria parasite—had been sequenced. The students, all in their twenties, said that the role of powerful computers and high-speed Internet access in making sense of the genome could not be overestimated. As the students sit in their laboratory at UCSD, mapping out the relationships between genes and proteins in *E. coli* and yeast, much of their raw data comes from the Internet, where full reports of various genome sequences and other experiments can be downloaded from public domain Web sites.

One striking example of the sheer amount of genomics data available to scientists on the Internet is that all 5.6 billion base pairs—As, Cs, Gs, and Ts—that have been sequenced in eukaryotic organisms can now be downloaded.

"When I first started this, I had no idea how complicated it was," said Timothy Allen, a 27-year-old Georgian using computing power and modeling to study patterns in DNA, with the goal of understanding how pathologies in the way DNA is packed may lead to disease. "You can just drown in the numbers. Even just a few years ago there was no way we could have done what we're doing now."

After visiting the labs of Palsson and Ideker, I was relieved to drop in on the graduate students of Professor Andrew McCulloch, whose work assumes a more tangible form. McCulloch specializes in the heart, unraveling its function from the genetic to the organ level. Under his tutelage, graduate students and postdocs—the workhorses in academic departments of biomedical engineering—spend their days doing everything from making computer models of rabbit hearts to trying to decode the workings of the fruit fly's cardiac genes.

McCulloch's lab is heir to the early biomedical engineering program at UCSD, when aeronautical engineer Y. C. Fung came to the university in 1964 and began collaborating closely with doctors and researchers at the medical school. At that time, the basic principles vital to aeronautical engineering—sheer stress, mechanics, air or fluid flow—were not being applied to medicine. Fascinated by the workings of the human body, Fung quickly grasped that many areas of physiology, such as cardiac function or air flow in lungs, could be better understood if viewed through the prism of engineering. He became an expert in pulmonary mechanics, and his successor, Shu Chien, is a leading researcher in cardiac mechanics.

"In my view, you don't understand things until you can write them down, express them mathematically, and predict them," said Fung, who, at age 85, regularly comes to his office at UCSD.

Although sixty-one years younger than Fung, Jake Feala is equally intrigued by the union of engineering and medicine. Feala's field of expertise is the fruit fly's heart, and when I visited with him, he was engaged in one of those tedious exercises of scientific investigation that may eventually yield a payoff. The fruit fly, *Drosophila melanogaster*, has 14,000 genes and one of the most primitive hearts in the insect world. Indeed, the fruit fly's heart is little more than a tube that pumps blood and lymphatic fluids to the insect's head and abdomen. When Feala placed one of the fruit flies under the microscope, its heart—working away at 350 beats per minute—bore a striking resemblance to the pulsating tube that I saw on the first ultrasound of my oldest daughter in utero fifteen years before. This is a major reason McCulloch is interested in the heart of the tiny insect, as it no doubt shares many cardiac genes with humans.

For his master's degree, Feala had taken on the mind-boggling task of examining 14,000 fruit flies, each with a different gene removed, or knocked out. One by one, he ran them under a microscope to examine their cardiac function. By comparing heart rates and the diameter of the heart tube, he planned to assemble a database of information on which genes, when knocked out, affected the hearts of fruit flies. His work is part of a larger effort to catalog the genes that affect the heart, in both fruit flies and humans, and to study their interactions.

"There are a lot of homologues between fruit flies and human beings," said Feala. "We want to come up with a nodule of closely connected genes related to cardiac function."

To accomplish his task, Feala, 24, called on his undergraduate training in biomedical and electrical engineering at the University of Wisconsin. He invented an ingenious device that sucked flies out of a tiny bottle and through a tube and—using an electric charge—pinned them on their back to a slide. He then wrote special software that traced the outline of the fly under a microscope and zeroed in on the heart, automatically tallying its rate and measuring its diameter. With this machine Feala invented what he called the first rapid, or "high throughput," method to compare genes and heart function in fruit flies.

I visited UCSD as his project was beginning and could not hide my amazement at the sheer magnitude of screening 14,000 fruit flies.

"We'll keep ordering the flies and do thousands of screenings," he told me. "I've always had fun designing things and making things. I like gadgets. Coming out of high school I really wanted to do something good for society. I thought about medical school. If you're a doctor, you can help one person at a time, but if you invent something worthwhile and develop a new technology, you could help millions of people."

Across the lab bench from Feala, graduate student Hunaid Gurji was working with a different kind of heart, this one from a rabbit. McCulloch's lab is nationally known for making computer models of hearts that could be used to analyze cardiac pathologies, such as heart failure, and which drugs might be used to treat them. Working with other graduate students, Gurji had sent the rabbit into heart failure by placing a cardiac pacemaker in the right ventricle and doubling the animal's heart rate, from about 180 beats per minute to 360. This rapid beating soon led to an inefficient pumping action, causing the heart to propel less blood into the body, retain more blood in the cardiac chambers, and grow steadily larger. After several weeks of this hyperactive pumping, the organ went into heart failure as the left ventricle expanded and its walls thinned.

On the day I visited Gurji, students had removed the heart from the rabbit and kept it beating by filling its left ventricle with a water-filled balloon. Gurji then painted forty reflective titanium oxide dots on the outside of the heart and injected it with a voltage-sensitive dye. He took pictures of the heart, using the reflective dots as a way to measure the forces and strain on various sections of the enlarged organ. He also used a pacemaker lead to send a wave of electricity through the heart, which was picked up by the voltage-sensitive dye and recorded by a special camera. The data from these tests, repeated on dozens of rabbits, were fed into a computer, which produced detailed, three-dimensional images showing the heart's flabby beat and its propensity to slide into arrhythmia. Such models are a good tool to devise therapies for treating heart failure, a common occurrence among humans whose cardiac tissue has been damaged by heart attack.

Other graduate students and postdoctoral fellows in McCulloch's lab are studying the heart on the cellular and genetic level. They are modeling how changes in the heart's chemistry can affect its mechanical function and, conversely, how changes in mechanics—after, say, a heart attack—affect cardiac chemistry. Some are studying how different levels of calcium, which plays a crucial role in causing heart cells and muscle to contract, affect cardiac function. Others are investigating the role of a crucial molecule—adenosine triphosphate (ATP)—in cardiac function. ATP is involved in the storage and transportation of energy between cells, and McCulloch's investigators are studying the link between heart disease and decreased ATP levels.

All this research, said McCulloch, is part of an effort to understand what makes the heart tick, from the lowest to the highest level.

"The heart is one of the very few systems where computational modeling has reached a high level," said McCulloch. "We're trying to connect these different levels of information, from molecules, to proteins, to cells, to tissues, and finally to the organ itself."

Further proof that, in the future, smaller is better in biomedical engineering can be seen in several labs at UCSD. Assistant Professor Sangeeta Bhatia is redefining tiny on several fronts. Like Martin Yarmush of Rutgers, she is interested in creating a bioartificial liver. One of the major hurdles is packing billions of cells into an engineered device, and this is where microtechnology comes into play. If Bhatia and others have any hope of re-creating the liver, they're going to have to rely on a series of minuscule, hivelike chambers. To accomplish that, researchers are devising three-dimensional, microfluidic chambers made in a similar way as computer processing chips. This involves taking a silicon wafer, using photolithography to burn miniature tunnels in the wafer, and then pouring silicon rubber over the wafer to form a channel half the width of a human hair.

In Bhatia's lab, graduate student Dave Eddington is helping create microfluidic chambers, one of which he showed me. On what looked like a small glass slide, I could see hundreds of lines looping back and forth, connected to two intake valves used to control the fluid flowing into the chamber. An important aspect of making an artificial liver that will function like a real one is the different gradients of blood-rich oxygen bathing hepatocytes. The gradient is dependent on how far cells are from the vessel-rich cores of the liver. Eddington believes that seeding liver cells into microfluidic chambers and then exposing them to varying blood oxygen levels will help sustain hepatocytes in artificial livers. In late 2004, Eddington succeeded in growing liver cells in his microfluidic chambers on the first try but then failed on two subsequent occasions. He was not discouraged.

"Biomedical engineering is so interesting to me because it is so immensely complicated," said Eddington. "We know so little now. The human body is the hardest thing to design engineering applications for."

At the University of California, Davis, Alexander Revzin, an assistant professor of biomedical engineering, is working on devices so tiny that he will be able to place 10,000 liver cells in 10,000 separate wells, all on a chip no more than one-eighth of an inch square. He achieves this through a technology called micropatterning, which involves shining a light onto photosensitive material to create 10,000 individual squares. The goal is to study all aspects of the cells' activity, including their gene expression and the proteins they make. Eventually, such a device could enable pharmaceutical companies to use micropatterned chips to perform rapid drug tests on cells from the liver and other tissues.

"My goal is to use microfabrication and nanotechnology to create an artificial environment and study hepatocytes under very controlled conditions," said Revzin. "One of my dreams is to have a microfabricated platform where different components of the cell environment are created, where I can take 5,000 or 10,000 liver cells, put them in a device, and have the cells influenced in ten different ways based on ten different conditions I create. I want to present single cells in a high-density format where they can be analyzed and extracted and you can do genomic research."

Revzin—a tall, powerfully built man whose family emigrated from Belarus to America in 1990—showed me a micropatterned surface, 1 millimeter square, containing 1,400 wells. Under a microscope, I could see individual cells sitting in wells that were one-fifth the diameter of a human hair. One way to get the cells to stick in such tiny spots is to treat the wells with different proteins, which helps retain cells in specific wells. Some neuroscientists and biomedical engineers are studying ways to attach neurons to micropatterned surfaces and then use those devices as a bridge to repair damaged nerves, such as the optical nerve connecting the eye to the brain. Other researchers are creating similarly tiny devices designed to slowly release drugs in targeted organs.

The ultimate in minuscule is nanotechnology, which is now the subject of intensive research at universities and laboratories around the world. Nanotechnology is based on the use of semiconductor crystals made of cadmium selenide, some approaching the incomprehensible size of a billionth of a meter. Depending on their size, nanotechnology crystals give off different colors and intensities of light, which makes them an ideal tool for imaging on the genetic and molecular level. The crystals also can be activated with light, electricity, or ultrasound, making them a potentially useful tool in delivering drug payloads.

Bhatia envisions using quantum dots—crystals less than 10 nanometers in diameter—as a kind of smart machine that can home in on the smallest workings of the cell. One potential use would be to locate and kill cancer cells.

"We want to design a multifunctional device that is an imaging agent, that can deliver a drug payload, and that can be interrogated with a radio frequency signal so it can report back to the doctor and say it's done its job," said Bhatia.

That goal may be years away, but Bhatia—working with Erikki Ruoslahti, an M.D./Ph.D. who is a distinguished professor at the Burnham Institute in La Jolla—is making progress. In 2002, Ruoslahti and Bhatia succeeded in attaching homing peptides, made up of nine amino acids, to quantum dots that targeted breast cancer cells in live mice. The quantum dots were injected intravenously, and the homing peptides guided the quantum dots to receptors on the breast cancer cells. Different homing peptides also directed the quantum dots to normal lung tissue and to the lymph nodes adjacent to breast cancer cells.

Austin Derfus, a Ph.D. student in Bhatia's lab, is investigating ways of attaching drugs to the quantum dots and then releasing the drugs directly at the site of a tumor using heat, ultrasound, or ultraviolet light. One long-term goal would be to blast drugs or genetic material directly into the nucleus of cancer cells to kill them.

Although still in its infancy, nanotechnology is a promising frontier, with the National Science Foundation predicting that this new realm of science could contribute $1 trillion to the U.S. economy by 2015.

The foray of biomedical engineers into the unknown territory of nanotechnology, genes, and stem cells seems, at this point, like an overwhelming challenge. But just half a century ago, numerous problems faced by medicine and engineering—safely pacing the heart or running it with a mechanical pump, imaging the body down to the finest detail, managing diabetes with insulin pumps—also appeared to pose nearly insurmountable difficulties. Those worlds have been substantially conquered. Now, biomedical engineers are focusing their attention on an entirely different universe, all the while displaying the same confidence that the mystery they're confronting is ultimately knowable and will inevitably yield to the onslaught of computers, mathematics, and science.

"These genetic networks are so complicated, and we really don't understand how they work," said Scott J. Bornheimer, a Ph.D. candidate in biochemistry who is studying under biomedical engineering professor Shankar Subramaniam. "It's like if you were an alien and you saw a car. You'd have no idea how it works. That's sort of the stage where we are now. We're trying to figure out what the parts are and how they fit together. In the end, it all comes back to solving problems. Right now there's a lot of exploration going on and not as much discovery. But I think it will all begin to come together soon, maybe in five or ten years, maybe longer."

Index

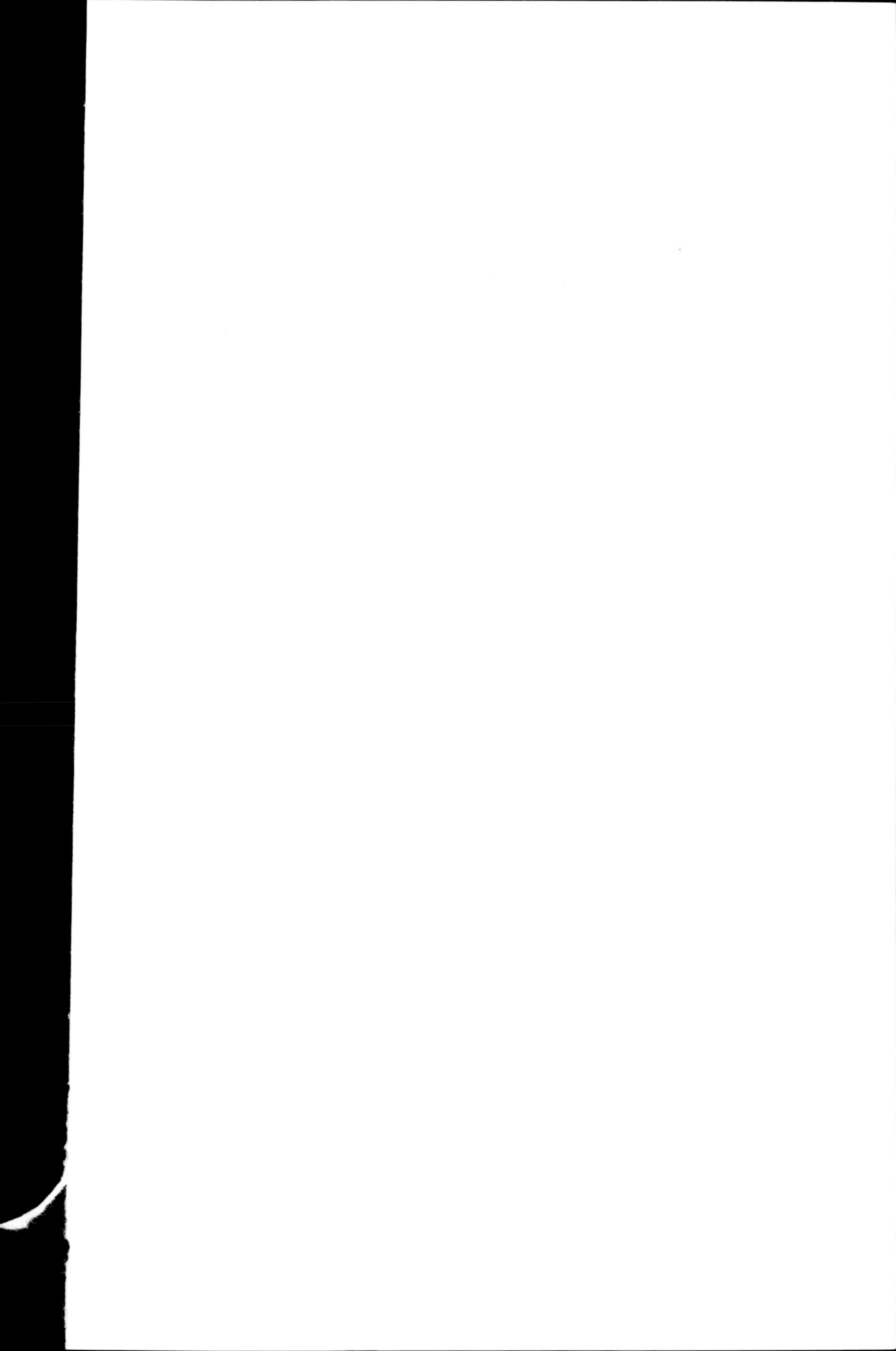